I0051109

Dwarfism, Spatiality and Disabling Experiences

This book provides an in-depth analysis of the social and spatial experiences of people with dwarfism, an impairment that results in a person being no taller than 4' 10".

This book engages with the concept that dwarfism's most prominent feature – body size and shape – can form the basis of social discrimination and disadvantages within society. By ignoring body size as a disability, it is hard to see the resulting disabling consequences of the built environment. Using a mixed-methods approach and drawing on the work undertaken by human geographers and disability studies academics, this book analyses how the relationship between harmful cultural stereotypes and space shapes everyday experiences of people with dwarfism and works to socially exclude them in diverse ways. Showing how spatial and social barriers are not mutually exclusive but can influence one another, this book responds to the limited academic work on the subject of dwarfism, whilst also contributing to the study of geographies of body size.

It will be of interest to all scholars and students of disability studies, human geography, the built environment, sociology and medical humanities.

Erin Pritchard is a lecturer in Disability and Education in the School of Social Sciences at Liverpool Hope University, UK.

Interdisciplinary Disability Studies
Series editor: Mark Sherry
The University of Toledo, USA

Disability studies has made great strides in exploring power and the body. This series extends the interdisciplinary dialogue between disability studies and other fields by asking how disability studies can influence a particular field. It will show how a deep engagement with disability studies changes our understanding of the following fields: sociology, literary studies, gender studies, bioethics, social work, law, education, or history. This ground-breaking series identifies both the practical and theoretical implications of such an interdisciplinary dialogue and challenges people in disability studies as well as other disciplinary fields to critically reflect on their professional praxis in terms of theory, practice, and methods.

Disability and Social Movements
Learning from Australian Experiences
Rachel Carling-Jenkins

Disability and Discourse Analysis
Jan Grue

Communication, Sport and Disability
The Case of Power Soccer
Michael S. Jeffress

Disability and Citizenship Studies
Marie Sépulchre

Women with Disabilities as Agents of Peace, Change and Rights
Experiences from Sri Lanka
Edited by Karen Soldatic and Dinesha Samararatne

Dwarfism, Spatiality and Disabling Experiences
Erin Pritchard

For a full list of titles in this series, please visit: www.routledge.com/Interdisciplinary-Disability-Studies/book-series/ASHSER1401

Dwarfism, Spatiality and Disabling Experiences

Erin Pritchard

Routledge
Taylor & Francis Group

LONDON AND NEW YORK

First published 2021
by Routledge
2 Park Square, Milton Park, Abingdon, Oxon OX14 4RN

and by Routledge
605 Third Avenue, New York, NY 10017

First issued in paperback 2022

Routledge is an imprint of the Taylor & Francis Group, an informa business

© 2021 Erin Pritchard

The right of Erin Pritchard to be identified as author of this work has been asserted by her in accordance with sections 77 and 78 of the Copyright, Designs and Patents Act 1988.

All rights reserved. No part of this book may be reprinted or reproduced or utilised in any form or by any electronic, mechanical, or other means, now known or hereafter invented, including photocopying and recording, or in any information storage or retrieval system, without permission in writing from the publishers.

Trademark notice: Product or corporate names may be trademarks or registered trademarks, and are used only for identification and explanation without intent to infringe.

Publisher's Note
The publisher has gone to great lengths to ensure the quality of this reprint but points out that some imperfections in the original copies may be apparent.

British Library Cataloguing-in-Publication Data
A catalogue record for this book is available from the British Library

Library of Congress Cataloging-in-Publication Data
Names: Pritchard, Erin, author.
Title: Dwarfism, spatiality and disabling experiences/Erin Pritchard.
Description: Milton Park, Abingdon, Oxon ; New York, NY : Routledge, 2021.
|Series: Interdisciplinary disability studies | Includes bibliographical references and index.
Identifiers: LCCN 2020029511 (print) | LCCN 2020029512 (ebook) | ISBN 9780367459062 (hardback) | ISBN 9781003026051 (ebook)
Subjects: LCSH: Dwarfism. | Metabolism--Disorders. | Dwarfism--Social aspects.
Classification: LCC RB140.3. P75 2021 (print) | LCC RB140.3 (ebook) | DDC 616.4/7--dc23
LC record available at https://lccn.loc.gov/2020029511
LC ebook record available at https://lccn.loc.gov/2020029512

ISBN 13: 978-0-367-64430-7 (pbk)
ISBN 13: 978-0-367-45906-2 (hbk)
ISBN 13: 978-1-00-302605-1 (ebk)

DOI: 10.4324/9781003026051

Typeset in Times New Roman
by MPS Limited, Dehradun

This book is dedicated to Kenneth Pritchard.

Contents

Acknowledgements

There are a number of people I would like to thank for helping me to complete this book.

First, thank you to all of the participants who took the time to share their thoughts and experiences with me. Without their contributions, this book would not have been possible. I am also grateful to my two doctoral supervisors, Prof Janice McLaughlin and Prof Peter Hopkins, who provided invaluable support and advice.

I am, of course, truly grateful to Prof Mark Sherry who gave me the initiative to write this book. Without his encouragement, I would never have thought that it could have been done. I am also grateful to Claire Jarvis for her support in getting this book going.

To my colleagues at Liverpool Hope University, I am very grateful and lucky to work with such a great bunch of people. I am especially grateful to Prof David Bolt for his continuous support and guidance. Thanks also to Jody Crutchley and Ella Houston for all of your encouragement.

Of course, I am very thankful to my family, Elaine Pritchard, Lee Pritchard, Thomas Pritchard, Laura Dekker and Marit Dekker. However, I am especially grateful to my dad, Kenneth Pritchard, who was a great support and fantastic company. I also must thank my friends, Laura Jane Pardoe, Ralitsa Hiteva, Stephanie Phillips and Lynne Freeman for continuous encouragement and support.

1 Introduction

1.1 Introduction

Dwarfism is a medical condition that results in a person being no taller than 4' 10" (Adelson, 2005a). Known medically as skeletal dysplasia (Shakespeare et al., 2007), there are over 200 different types of dwarfism with underlying impairments that often differ. Spinal stenosis, for example, is mostly associated with a form of dwarfism known as Achondroplasia. Depending on the type of dwarfism, a person's body is either disproportionate or proportionate in size. People with dwarfism who are proportionate appear only to be small in stature; their arms, legs, trunk and head are in the same proportion as an average-size person. Examples of proportionate dwarfism include primordial dwarfism. People with dwarfism whose bodies are disproportionate have a torso of average size but short arms and legs. Achondroplasia is an example of disproportionate dwarfism and is the most common form of dwarfism. It is estimated that approximately 250,000 people have Achondroplasia worldwide (Horton et al., 2007). The cause of Achondroplasia is genetic.

This book revolves around dwarfism's most prominent feature—body size and shape. It engages with a social constructivist understanding of disability to demonstrate the social implications of having a body size which does not meet society's standard. The social model of disability argues that disability is the result of a society that does not take into account the needs of disabled people, and thus physical structures lead to inaccessibility (Oliver, 1990). This book shows that people with dwarfism are disabled through unaccommodating public spaces, which do not take into account the small body. It explores the spatial barriers people with dwarfism encounter due to their small stature and how they deal with these barriers. This book aims to create a broader understanding of the social and spatial experiences of people with dwarfism, whilst attempting to respond to some of the misconceptions about dwarfism, including its contention as a disability. This book contributes to both Social geographies and Disability studies, showing how a bodily difference, which is predominantly about height, is disabled by a 'one size fits all society'. As disability can be understood as a social construct, applying a geographical perspective can aid in further understanding how the built environment is disabling for people with impairments.

Geographies of disability consist of a diverse range of research which explores the socio-spatial experiences of disability (Butler and Bowlby, 1997; 1999a; Chouinard et al., 2010; Dyck, 1995, 1999; Edwards, 2013; Crooks et al., 2008; Hall, 2004, 2007, 2010, 2011; Hall and Kearns, 2001; Gleeson, 1997, 1999a, 1999b, 2000; Hahn, 1986, 1996; Hawksworth, 2001; Imrie, 1996a, 1996b, 1999, 2000, 2004, 2012; Imrie and Edwards, 2007; Imrie and Hall, 2001; Kitchin, 1998; Kitchin and Law, 2001; Moss, 1999; Moss and Dyck, 1996; Parr, 1997; Parr et al., 2004; Philo, 2005; Philo et al., 2005; Worth, 2013). Adopting the views of Mike Oliver (1990), Gleeson (1997, 1999a, 1999b) argues that disability is the result of industrialisation within western societies, which includes inaccessible buildings and transport systems, as well as devaluing cultural imagery. Kitchin (1998) argues that it is important to recognise the role of space in reproducing and maintaining disabled people's exclusion from the built environment. Soja (1989) argues that space is a social product and shaping force in social life.

The book uses the term 'socio-spatial' barrier throughout. Space is a structure, but with addition of the term 'socio' it becomes a social product (Soja, 1989). The French Sociologist Henri Lefebvre (1991) is credited with the idea that spaces are socially produced. According to Lefebvre (1991:289), '(social) space is a (social) product'. The social production of a space is important to consider as it helps us to explore how spaces are created in a way that does not take into account people with dwarfism and thus means that they will experience the built environment differently to other people.

According to Lefebvre space can be conceived as a triad, which contains representations of spaces, representational space and spatial practice in order to understand how spaces are socially produced. Lefebvre (1991) suggests that representations of space are conceived spaces designed by planners. The representations of space influence the meaning and materiality of a space. The materiality is associated with the physical structure of a space, whilst the meaning is associated with how it will be used and by whom. How a space is conceived by planners can impact the spatial practice of different users. The spatial practice relates to how people negotiate and use different spaces. Representational space relates to the meaning of that space to the user, which in turn also impacts people's spatial practice.

A spatial barrier is physically inaccessible and using the addition of the term 'socio' can be seen as a barrier created by ableist planners and architects who do not take into account the needs of people with dwarfism. This in turn leads to disabling situations, impacting the spatial practice of people with dwarfism. These disabling situations become entwined with social interactions when people with dwarfism have to ask for help or draw attention to themselves when interacting with a space differently. The word barrier can also be taken to mean obstacle—obstacles that can either restrict access or be overcome somehow. A barrier does not necessarily mean that a person encounters a physical barrier and therefore it cannot always be overcome; it just inhibits a person's use of a space or particular facility.

How we experience spaces is dependent on our identity. Massey (1994: 3) suggests that, 'the social relations of space are experienced differently, and variously interpreted, by those holding different positions as part of it'. This is where it is important to introduce the notion of ableism. According to Chouinard *ableism* is 'a set of ideas, practices, institutions and social relations that presume ablebodieness and by doing so constructs persons with disabilities as marginalised and largely invisible others'. In relation to dwarfism, ableism is constructed by heightism and has existed for centuries. *Heightism* can be defined as a form of discrimination experienced by people whose height deviates significantly from the norm. As tall stature is revered within society, people with dwarfism are likely to experience heightism in different forms, such as having to interact with spaces that are not size suitable for them.

As spaces are a social product, then it is fair to say that they are created for the non-disabled person, which impacts how disabled people interact and navigate through these spaces. In relation to dwarfism, Kruse (2002, 2010) argues that spaces are 'statuarized', in other words designed for the average-sized person. This impacts how people with dwarfism interact and navigate through spaces. The statuarization of spaces can be applied to both the meaning and materiality of them. According to Kruse (2002), spaces are physically constructed to suit the average-sized person (materiality) and contain messages that encourage tallness to be revered (meaning). In consideration of spaces being statuarized, it is also important to explore work within geographies of body size.

Within Social Geography, the subject of body size is now gaining momentum with a growing body of research which focuses on how the sized body interacts with and experiences spaces (Colls, 2004, 2006; Evans et al., 2012; Hopkins, 2012; Longhurst, 2005, 2010). As representations of spaces are based upon the average-sized person, then it is important to understand the spatial practices of body sizes that exceed the norm. Drawing upon theories within Disability studies, Geographies of body size recognise the spatial barriers for people who are not of average size. By understanding different spatial relations, we can explore how different spaces are disabling for people with dwarfism. This relates to the notion of normalcy and how the construction of spaces results in disabling experiences for those whose body size deviates from the norm. Overall, it is suggested that disability is a product of society and not a person's bodily difference, and thus disability can be reduced or eliminated through taking into account the needs of various impairments as well as challenging attitudes.

1.2 Aims and objectives

The book explores a number of key questions concerned with the social and spatial barriers experienced by people with dwarfism within public spaces:

- How do people with dwarfism negotiate spatial barriers in the context of unaccommodating structures?
- What social responses do people with dwarfism experience when dealing with spatial barriers within public spaces?
- Do people with dwarfism avoid certain spaces in order to avoid negative social situations?
- Do resources which are nominally called 'accessible' help or hinder people with dwarfism in their negotiation of public spaces?
- How do people with dwarfism feel that cultural representations of dwarfism affect society's treatment towards them?

There are a number of elements which can affect how people experience different spaces. In relation to dwarfism, it is important to consider some spatial practices which are unique to them. For example, it is not expected for the non-disabled person to interact with a space differently, as that space has been created with the notion that they can carry out a task in the way expected, due to the way that space has been constructed. However, as most spaces will not have been created for people with dwarfism, their spatial practices will differ. This book explores the social barriers people with dwarfism encounter when dealing with spatial barriers, providing a transition from the spatial to the social, and showing how one can possibly lead to the other. Additionally, by including 'accessible' spaces and facilities within a discussion of dwarfism and disability, the book problematises the idea that such spaces are always a suitable option for people with dwarfism.

In order to gain a deeper understanding of such social experiences, this book questions the role of cultural representations of dwarfism and whether they contribute to how they are perceived within society that could lead to social barriers. Dwarfism is saturated in cultural baggage that includes harmful stereotypes, deeply affecting the rights and social experiences of people with dwarfism. Most people will have never met someone with dwarfism, but will recall seeing them in some form of entertainment, which shapes how they perceive them. According to Haller (2010), people's perceptions of disabled people are largely media-driven. These perceptions are constructed by ableist representations of dwarfism that have been around for centuries. Ablon (1990) points out that dwarfism is a physically distinctive and easily recognisable impairment and thus seeing a person with dwarfism in public is likely to provoke a reaction. This book is particularly interested in what spaces and situations such reactions occur within. It argues that the implications of such reactions result in psycho-emotional disablism that influence the way a person with dwarfism negotiates different spaces.

1.3 Motivation and justification

My motivation for writing this book is both personal and academic. I have dwarfism, and throughout my life I have experienced numerous social and spatial barriers. I have come to realise that I navigate spaces differently. For example, I often avoid spaces that I know to be inaccessible or where I am likely to receive unwanted attention, evident in past experiences of that space or just from observing the space and its occupants. Shakespeare et al. (2010) suggest that people with dwarfism often avoid locations where they receive unwanted attention. It is easier than dealing with the unwanted attention from average-sized people and their children, especially when trying to counteract negative attitudes usually results in more abuse.

My Achondroplasia does not only cause short stature but has a number of other secondary impairments, including spinal stenosis which causes both pain and mobility impairments. However, I find that the biggest obstacles that I encounter are related to society's response to my short stature. Additionally, I am often told that I am 'not disabled' by people who barely know me. They state that I can walk, so they ask how can I be disabled? Yet they do not see me struggle using an ATM, high counters, and having to have my car adapted to be able to drive like them. The dirty looks I get for walking to my car parked in the disabled bay continue, despite the pain brought on by my spinal stenosis, or having to carry shopping bags weighing me down because the shopping trolley is too big for me to use.

I have also grown up and seen people with dwarfism in various forms of media and noticed that because of their dwarfism, the way they are represented is often harmful and inaccurate. They are never shown as fully human or as someone experiencing the realities of dwarfism. I felt that the rarity of dwarfism, coupled with such misrepresentations, means people fail to see the disabling experiences associated with dwarfism. My identity is constructed by strangers who rely on misrepresentations, often leading me to be ridiculed and mocked. The audiences would see people with dwarfism running around and making fools of themselves, but they would never see people with dwarfism within society struggling to walk or being angry because they were unable to do something as simple as posting a letter. I wanted to know what other experiences people with dwarfism had and if I could bring them together in order to make them visible to a wider audience.

My other motivation for writing is academic. There is a limited amount of literature available on the lives of people with dwarfism, with a few exceptions, such as where they are featured in books focusing on human oddities and freaks (Adelson, 2005a). These books usually contain a number of images of people with dwarfism from the early Victorian era, such as Charles Stratton, aka 'General Tom Thumb', who was often paraded around for people to see, including Queen Victoria. These kinds of books provide a way of allowing the reader to stare at people with bodily abnormalities whilst providing very little understanding about their everyday lives. I flicked through one of these books as a child and although I shared an impairment with some of the people featured in them, I could not relate to them. They somehow seemed exotic and not part of society. What I did not realise at the time was that I was being exposed to an ableist representation of dwarfism, which impacted how I viewed dwarfism and accepted my own impairment.

As well as people with dwarfism being represented as freaks or oddities, Kruse (2003) suggests that there is very little academic research that focuses on the social aspects of dwarfism, rather research tends to focus on the medical side of the impairment. Thompson et al. (2008) review the current literature available in relation to the medical, health and social aspects of dwarfism and suggest that not only is research limited, but is often unreliable. This is because of an over-emphasis on the experiences of children with dwarfism; there are few books which give an insight into the lives of adults with dwarfism. This book will engage with the limited, yet important, literature on adults with dwarfism, but is groundbreaking because of its applied and interdisciplinary focus that combines Social Geography and Disability studies. I want to show people with dwarfism as everyday people as opposed to oddities, adding to the limited academic literature that focuses on the everyday lives of adults with dwarfism.

To gather the data used in this book, a qualitative methodology relying on semi-structured interviews which incorporated photo elicitation exercises was adopted. Photo elicitation exercises were added to understand how people with dwarfism experience public spaces and why they may navigate them differently. Twenty-two interviews, mostly with women with dwarfism living in the UK, were conducted between 2009–2010. These interviews allowed the participants to share their views and experiences with me. Participants were recruited through associations for people with dwarfism, groups for people with dwarfism on the social networking site Facebook and through snowball sampling. All participants have been given pseudonyms for confidentiality reasons. Any demographic information mentioned in the book has also been made vague; for example, instead of mentioning the exact town or city the participant lives in, a vague description is given, such as the 'North west of England'.

1.4 Terminology

I consider the choice of words I use in this book to be important, as language can affect not only how disability and dwarfism is understood but also can have different meanings to different people. The language we use influences and reflects our understanding of the social world (Barnes and Mercer, 2010). In relation to dwarfism, there is a lot of contention and confusion in relation to the correct name given to an impairment. This can be frustrating as the lack of understanding and agreement upon what term should be used to refer to a person with dwarfism often allows more problematic terms to be used. For example, the term 'midget' is an offensive term, which this book will show. However, I often come across it being used freely within the media and by people who are unaware of its offense. I would like to hope that this book can help to clear up some confusion and aid in coming to an agreement on what terms are acceptable or unacceptable. Therefore, I first want to justify why I have chosen to use the term 'people with dwarfism' to refer to people who all have various forms of dwarfism.

When conducting the research for this book, it was apparent that the participant's preferred name for their impairment ranged from person with dwarfism, dwarf, person with restricted growth, person of short stature and little person. Some participants liked the term 'dwarf' and disliked 'little person', while others preferred 'restricted growth' but did not like 'dwarf' and so on. The term 'dwarf' is the most common term used both medically and socially when referring to someone with dwarfism. Despite this, some people contest the use of the word 'dwarf' due to its relation to mythology. This is why 'person with dwarfism' has been chosen for this book, as it demonstrates that these are people with a specific impairment. It also leaves room for other identities, such as their gender or nationality, whereas 'dwarf' overshadows them.

Similarly, the term 'dwarf' and its connection to the mythic, little person can be used to refer to a Leprechaun or a child (Adelson, 2005b). The term 'little person' which was coined by the association 'Little People of America,' is very popular in the US but less so in the UK. Although 'little person' was preferred by some participants, it could not only refer to a child, but just someone of short stature who is not necessarily under 4' 10" (147 cm) and possibly does not have any underlying impairments, or in most cases, a disproportionate body size. In regards to 'restricted growth' and 'short stature', these terms could also refer to someone who is just short and not a person who has any of the impairments known collectively as dwarfism. This is problematic as something I wish to avoid is the assumption that people who are just small know what it is like to have dwarfism. I am often told by people who are 5' (152 cm) that they know what it is like to be a 'dwarf'. This I find problematic, as their assumption can dilute the disabling experiences of dwarfism. To try to shut them down; I will ask them how much they paid for their car's pedal extensions or if they have ever been asked if they do 'panto'. Of course, it is not to ignore that people who are short do not experience heightism, but that there are experiences unique to people with dwarfism, which often remain unknown.

In relation to disability, terminology is contested and terms usually vary between 'people with disabilities' and 'disabled people' (Shildrick, 2012). When referring to disability in general, this book has chosen to use the term 'disabled people' rather than 'people with disabilities'. A person does not have a disability, but rather is disabled by external factors. Morris (2001) points out that the term 'disability' does not refer to a person's impairment but rather prejudice and discrimination within society which is aimed at people with impairments. The term 'disabled people' is now considered more acceptable because people with impairments are disabled by society, not by their bodies (Shakespeare, 2006). As this book adopts a social constructivist understanding of disability; the term 'disabled people' is more appropriate to use.

1.5 Outline of chapters

This book is divided into four main analysis chapters and an overall conclusion. Each analysis chapter focuses on a different spatial experience, which put altogether should aid in providing a deep understanding of how people with dwarfism experience public spaces. Chapter 2, *Access tall areas*, explores how people with dwarfism have to negotiate a built environment created for the average-sized person. Public spaces are not size-suitable for people with dwarfism, creating disabling situations which influence how they navigate the built environment. Placing such experiences within the context of literature that critically analyses notions of 'normalcy' and drawing on the social model of disability, the chapter highlights the ways in which public spaces become sites of marginalisation and discrimination. For instance, public buildings and public transport are not fully accessible for people with dwarfism. To navigate such disabling barriers, people with dwarfism engage in a range of strategies, including the avoidance of particular spaces.

Chapter 2 also discusses the ways in which supposedly accessible spaces created for disabled people can be both enabling and disabling for people with dwarfism. The discussion engages notions of disability, including cultural imagery, which shapes the representation of disabled spaces. Engaging with UK disability policies and legislation, in particular Part M of the Buildings and Regulations Act (2010), the chapter demonstrates how these policies often ignore the needs of people with dwarfism. The last section of the chapter discusses how spaces and facilities designed for children can also be enabling or disabling due to their construction. One concern is that these spaces can result in disablist infantilization. If a space is made to accommodate children (for example, some places have separate washroom facilities for children), then it is likely to be accessible for people with dwarfism, however, it remains associated with children. Similarly, if a resource is purposely put out of reach to prevent a child from accessing it, then a person with dwarfism will also be unable to reach it. This not only creates a disabling situation, but it also infantilizes them as they are left in the same situation as a child. These understandings of spaces help to lead on to how people with dwarfism react towards spatial barriers, which are influenced by social attitudes within particular spaces.

Chapter 3, *Resisting spaces*, focuses on how people with dwarfism deal with spatial barriers either through dependency or navigating/overcoming the barrier in their own way. This chapter explores how these forms of resistance to an inaccessible built environment are not straightforward but are impacted by social attitudes. For example, some people with dwarfism may choose not to utilize a resource because doing something differently can generate unwanted attention such as staring or mockery. This is where the notion of psycho-emotional disablism is introduced, as unwanted attention can impact upon their well-being. This shows how access issues are also deeply connected with social barriers. Spatial barriers and social barriers are not mutually exclusive; one can lead to another. Likewise, issues of dependency are not straightforward but are also associated with more general perceptions of people with dwarfism.

Chapter 4, *Disabling identities*, discusses the contentious question of whether dwarfism should be recognised as a disability as opposed to a bodily difference. Unlike other impairments, people with dwarfism often remain absent from representations of disability, which hides the numerous barriers they encounter within different spaces. Drawing on research within Geographies of body size, this chapter explores people with dwarfism's perception of 'dwarfism as a disability' and helps the reader to gain a better understanding of what disability is. This part argues that people with dwarfism often deny themselves a disabled identity due to internalised ableism. This internalised ableism, it is argued, is constructed by social attitudes about disability and dwarfism.

The chapter then focuses on how the contention surrounding dwarfism as a disability leads to discussions of how people with dwarfism negotiate the built environment. In the first part of this chapter, social interactions between people with dwarfism and other members of the public are explored, particularly concerning instances where people with dwarfism try to access accessible spaces. This discussion adds to understanding of how people with dwarfism deal with spatial barriers and how they can be hindered by social barriers that are formed by people's understanding of disability. It argues that these interactions result in unequal power relations.

This analysis adds to previous work concerning how people with invisible impairments are challenged when trying to access accessible spaces. However, what this chapter also helps to show is that an impairment does not necessarily have to be invisible, it just does not have to meet a stereotypical perception of disability. Moving on, the second part of the chapter explores how attitudes change when people with dwarfism use a mobility scooter or wheelchair and thus take on the role of a differently disabled person. This part of the chapter exposes a hierarchy of disability, which is formed by representations of dwarfism and disability. This helps to lead onto the next chapter, which explores cultural representations of people with dwarfism.

Chapter 5, *Cultural representations of Dwarfism and their social consequences*, highlights the strong link between the entertainment industry and dominant understandings of dwarfism. The entire social experience of dwarfism, including the navigation of public space, is profoundly wrapped in the negative cultural representations, including those promulgated by the entertainment industry. And yet such negative images of dwarfism also have a long history. This chapter will provide an overview of how people with dwarfism have been culturally represented and argue that cultural representations of people with dwarfism are constructed by ableism, which perceives the non-normative body as inferior. Unlike other accounts of such harmful cultural representations, however, this chapter enables people with dwarfism to reflect on the ways the effects of these forms of representation affect their lives. Everyone is familiar with dwarfism in culture, but few people understand how this affects people with dwarfism in society. This chapter provides a voice to people with dwarfism that shows how they think dwarfism has been represented and what implications this has for them within society, including from name-calling to being physically manhandled. Using the agenda-setting theory (Shaw, 1979), this chapter shows how cultural representations of dwarfism influence how society perceives and interacts with them. Of course, this can affect how people with dwarfism negotiate public spaces, such as by avoiding particular spaces. Again, this demonstrates how spaces are socially produced to exclude certain bodies. It also further engages with the views of people with dwarfism on how they think dwarfism can be better represented in order to improve social encounters.

Chapter 6, *The politics of space, identity and the sized body*, draws the book to a conclusion. It summarizes the main themes such as dwarfism and the politics of space, dwarfism and disability identities, dwarfism and geographies of the body, dwarfism, the social model and disability studies, the significance of avoidance and challenging cultural representations of dwarfism. The chapter provides recommendations on improving equality for people with dwarfism in society, including exploring how Universal Design can be used as a more inclusive design approach for disabled people, as well as encouraging more positive cultural representations of people with dwarfism to improve social encounters.

2 Access tall spaces

2.1 Introduction

All public spaces and the facilities within them, from door handles to supermarket checkouts, are purposely created to be ergonomically suitable for the average-sized person. Ergonomics is defined as, 'the study of the problems of people in adjusting to their environment; the science that seeks to adapt work to working conditions to suit the user' (Panero and Zelnik, 1979: 313). The measurements of these spaces and the facilities within them are based on specific anthropometrics. Anthropometrics is derived from the Greek word '*anthropos*', meaning 'human', and '*metron*', meaning 'measure' (Panero and Zelnik, 1979). These measurements ensure that the average-sized person can easily interact with these facilities. This means that people with dwarfism have to interact with spaces and facilities that are not size suitable for them. This chapter unpacks the various socio-spatial barriers that people with dwarfism encounter on a daily basis.

As their experiences are influenced by their stature, the subject of body size is important to consider. Hopkins (2008, 2012) suggests that 'understanding how people negotiate everyday spaces, which are planned for specific bodies, is crucial in advancing the knowledges of geographies of body size'. The purpose of this chapter is to explore how people with dwarfism negotiate public spaces and understand how spaces can be both disabling and enabling depending on how they are designed and constructed. It demonstrates how spaces are '*statuarized*', a term coined by the US Social Geographer Rob Kruse (2002, 2010). According to Kruse (2002), spaces are physically constructed to suit the average-sized person and contain messages that encourage tallness to be revered. Engaging with spaces beyond those created for the average-sized, able-bodied person demonstrates how different spaces are enabling or disabled for people with dwarfism, depending on their statuarization. These different spaces include accessible spaces created for disabled people and spaces created for children.

First, this chapter focuses on how different spaces and facilities, including public transport, form socio-spatial barriers for people with dwarfism. It also explores the range of practices people with dwarfism use to negotiate socio-spatial barriers, including overcoming them in their own way, accessing alternative spaces or avoiding spaces. Second, the chapter explores how accessible spaces can be both enabling and disabling depending on how they have been constructed and for whom. It questions whether accessible spaces are accommodating for people with dwarfism by drawing on disability access policies and the participant's own experiences. Finally, it focuses on how spaces and the facilities within them which are adapted for children can be both enabling or disabling for people with dwarfism, depending on their purpose. Overall this chapter demonstrates how people with dwarfism are not considered when implementing a variety of spaces, which renders them out of place.

2.2 Disability, normalcy and people with dwarfism

How disability is understood is important to consider in order to understand how disabled people, or more specifically people with dwarfism, navigate the built environment. Whilst society in general often views disability as a medical condition, in Disability studies it is understood as a social phenomenon:

> Over the past forty years, disability has been argued to be a social phenomenon, created by different social processes. This conflicts with medical notions of disability, which places it upon the person. In 1975, the Union of the Physically Impaired Against Segregation (UPIAS) published the Fundamental Principles of Disability (UPIAS, 1975). The document made a distinction between impairment and disability. It argued that impairment was not the cause of disability, but rather "it is society which disables physically impaired people" (UPIAS, 1975: 3).

Using this concept of disability, UPIAS came up with the following definitions that separated impairment and disability:

> **Impairment:** lacking part or all of a limb, or having a defective limb, organism or mechanism of the body.

> **Disability:** the disadvantage or restriction of activity caused by a contemporary social organisation which takes no or little account of people who have physical impairments and thus excludes them from the mainstream of social activities (UPIAS, 1975: 3–4).

Focusing on the definition of impairment, it does not quite cover dwarfism as an impairment, as well as other impairments, including learning disabilities. Although dwarfism can result in joint and spinal problems, which can be related to having a 'defective mechanism of the body', the definition does not include body size as an impairment, unless you take defective limb to mean a limb or limbs not being of average size, which could partially cover some forms of dwarfism.

Understanding disability as a product of society indicates that it is also through changes in society that disability can be reduced or eliminated. Oliver (2004) states that disability can be understood in terms of two models: the medical model of disability and the social model of disability. The medical model of disability considers disability to be a medical problem that resides in the individual as a defect of the body that needs fixing through medical intervention in order to function within society (Oliver, 2004). This understanding of disability suggests that the person's body needs to be changed in order to meet society's expectations and thus be able to function within a society created for the 'general' population. Shakespeare (1996: 95) states that, 'the medical model of disability focuses on physical difference and that disabled people are classed as a group of people whose bodies do not work; or look different or act differently; or cannot do productive work'.

The social model of disability is mostly associated with British perspectives on impairments and disability and has been one of the key concepts within Disability studies. The main goal of the social model is to provide increased inclusion within society, including improved access to the built environment. It is not only used in academia but also as a political tool to promote positive changes within society for disabled people, including the implementation of disability-related policies and legislation, including the Disability Discrimination Act (1995). The social model of disability takes the focus away from the person and instead places it onto society and the disabling barriers it imposes upon disabled people (Oliver, 2004). The social model of disability argues that disability is created through the exclusion of people with impairments from capitalist production (Abberley, 1997; Barnes, 1991a; Finkelstein, 1980; and Oliver, 1990) and thus can be considered a Marxist materialist approach to understanding disability. Political economy, which Marxism is a part of, suggests that all phenomena, including disability, are produced by the economic and social forces of capitalism (Oliver, 1994). It suggests that during industrialisation within western societies, disabled people were deemed unproductive and unable to contribute to the accumulation of capital. Disabled people were therefore excluded from society, often through being placed in workhouses or institutions and in some cases freak shows. Social model writers suggest that the social position of disabled people continues to be primarily a product of the effects of the economic organisation of society and the requirements of capitalism. Gleeson (1999) argues that disabling spaces are a product of capitalist societies that result in disabled people experiencing numerous socio-spatial barriers. These socio-spatial barriers include inaccessible buildings, housing and transport systems, and are a result of how spaces are conceived. Imrie (1996) blames architects and planners for creating an inaccessible environment that discriminates against people with impairments, creating social inequalities. As Imrie (2004: 281) states: ... 'there is a tendency for architects to design and construct spaces to specific technical standards and dimensions, which revolve around the conception of the "normal" body, creating physical barriers for anyone who does not fit the conception of the normal body.'

These dimensions include the average stature of a person, resulting in disablement for people with dwarfism. Imrie (1996b) often refers to the ideas of Le Corbusier's 'Modular' conception of the normal body which is a person approximately six feet in height (183 cm), taunt, strong and showing no signs of physical or mental impairments. 'Modular' became a device to enable architects to create spaces and buildings based on the scale of a human being. This scale is based on averages. According to Lefebvre (1991), the ways spaces are perceived and produced are dependent on the occupant of that space. If spaces are perceived to be predominantly for the average-sized, able-bodied person, then spaces will be constructed to suit them. This is also true of accessible spaces, except they will be constructed to suit society's perception of a typical disabled person.

The idea of creating spaces for the average person relates to particular conceptions of normalcy. The concept of 'normalcy', unlike that of 'the ideal', implies that the majority of the population must or should somehow be part of the norm. The concept of the 'norm' demonstrates how the majority creates the average: it relies on the majority of the population falling under the arch of the standard bell-shaped curve. According to Davis (2006: 5), 'the average man, the body of the man in the middle, becomes the exemplar of the middle way of life'. The use of the average man can be related to the notion of ableism. Ableism is described as 'denoting an attitude that devalues or differentiates disability through the valuation of able-bodiedness equated to normalcy' (Campbell, 2009: 5). People with dwarfism exceed the norm and subsequently possess devalued traits (small body and in most cases a disproportionate body size), which are deemed undesirable within society.

In terms of height, an average can be calculated by measuring the height of the population. Of course, people with dwarfism will end up being an extreme deviation of this average. Those that deviate from the bell curve the most are considered extremities and are often undesirable. Whilst height is strongly constructed by the notion of normalcy and therefore heights that deviate in extremes from the norm are considered undesirable, they are rarely considered as disabling. This can have implications for people with dwarfism accessing accessible spaces.

2.3 Accessing and avoiding 'Tall' spaces

A common disabling barrier for people with dwarfism are high counters, which are found in a variety of public places including cafés, banks and post offices. High counters are difficult to see over due to the height of the counter as they are constructed on the presumption that a person will be tall enough to see over them when standing up. Not being able to see over a counter makes it difficult to carry out tasks in the way expected:

Michelle: *The counters are sometimes high, and sometimes when you are in a queue they [staff] don't see you and instead serve the person behind you.*

Michelle is unable to fully interact in that space and leaves her out of place, both spatially and socially. Imrie and Kumar (1998) suggest that high barriers cause invisibility for disabled people. The problem may at first be the high barrier, which causes their invisibility, but this also creates a social barrier. In both cases, Michelle experiences disablism, as her inability to get served is an infringement on her equal access to the built environment. The construction of public spaces allows the dominant group within society, which in this case is people of average stature, to be able to fully interact effectively in spaces with limited disruption, reflecting an ableist situation. Being unable to see over a high counter in one space causes a disabling situation, causing a person to navigate through the built environment differently by finding a more accessible space:

Amanda: *If I know a place has a high counter or something and another one down the road does not then, I will go to the other.*

Amanda shows resistance to a disabling space by finding a place that is accessible to her. An inaccessible public space causes disabled people to confine their activities to locations that are relatively barrier free (Hahn, 1986). Limiting the places a person can access is a form of social exclusion as the person does not have the same level of access as other members of the public. This lack of choice reflects disablism as the disabled person is confined to a certain space.

People with dwarfism encounter a number of spatial barriers when supermarket shopping, including when packing and paying for items at the checkout:

Joan and Steve: *Some of the checkouts are quite high, and also with the shopping you are doing your own packing, and they just shove the stuff down the end of the checkout, and they put it quite far over so you can't reach it. I have to keep asking them to move it over to us.*

Joan and Steve, a married couple who both have dwarfism, do their shopping together but find packing their shopping at the checkout difficult due to its height and size. Typical checkouts have a large area at the end, where the customers' items go after being scanned. This area is surrounded by a small barrier in order to prevent items from falling off. A person needs to be tall enough and have an average-sized arm length in order to be able to reach over the barrier, take their items and place them into their shopping bag or trolley. In order to overcome this problem Joan and Steve are reliant on the cashier understanding their needs. The cashier's understanding of their needs is not always apparent, which exacerbates the disabling situation. A more accessible facility and better staff awareness is required in order to allow people with dwarfism an easier shopping experience. In most spaces there is a lack of accessible checkouts, however, more supermarkets are providing checkouts that provide choices for the independent, non-disabled customer.

In many supermarkets, across the UK, self-service checkouts are now available. According to Petrie et al. (2014), in neoliberal societies, self-service facilities are becoming more common. Self-service checkouts are an alternative to the regular checkouts, allowing consumers to scan and bag their own items as well as pay directly for their items using the facility's inbuilt till. When shown an image of a self-service checkout, the majority of participants spoke about how these checkouts were difficult or impossible to use due to different parts of the facility, such as the item scanner and touch screen, being out of reach as Naomi explains:

Naomi: *I despise those [self-service checkouts]. I find them too high. I am not very good with lifting stuff above my shoulders which is very low. I often can't see the screens. They are not clear when you are lower as they are usually wide-angle screens. When you look up, the screen is usually dark, because the contrast isn't good from a wide angle. I find getting the chip and pin machine down very awkward and then also having to cover your pin is difficult. I don't like self-service machines at all.*

Instead of a suitable alternative being created for disabled people, an alternative has been provided which only benefits non-disabled people who are already able to use the regular checkouts without any perceived difficulties. Petrie et al. (2014) point out that suppliers of self-service checkouts are often reluctant to consider the access needs of disabled customers as they are concerned about the additional costs required to provide accessible self-service checkouts. The reason for the self-service checkout is economics, as they create increased profits for the supermarkets by reducing the number of staff they employ because one member of staff can manage several self-service checkouts. The economic advantages for the supermarkets override the needs of people with dwarfism. It is important to recognise that people with dwarfism are not only disabled by the height of the facility, but also by being expected to lift items that they must scan. Not only is Naomi unable to use the self-service checkout, but being unable to cover her pin number also demonstrates a security issue as people will be able to see her bank details, which places her in a vulnerable situation.

Another disabling situation is created within a supermarket when using a shopping trolley. Supermarkets are equipped with various trolleys, including a deep trolley for people wanting to do a large shop, a shallow trolley for a lighter shop, a handbasket for when buying a few essentials and an accessible trolley which can be fitted onto a wheelchair. It can be noted that within most supermarkets there are a range of trolleys available but this range, as all participants pointed out, is limited as all trolleys are not size suitable for them. Many of the participants spoke about not using the deep trolleys because the depth and height of the trolley made them difficult or impossible to use:

Amanda: *I can only use the shallow trolleys, the deep trolleys are impossible to use as I can't get any of my shopping out as the trolley is too big.*

Most shopping trolleys are over three feet in height, making them too high for the majority of people with dwarfism to use. The alternative to using a deep trolley was using a shallow trolley, although, as Charlotte mentions, they are not always available:

Charlotte: *Those big ones [trolleys] are ridiculous, they are impossible. What annoys me at times is that they sometimes run out of the shallow ones which I use and so I can't do my shopping. I can't get things out of the big trolleys.*

When other members of the public are shopping, they are given a choice of trolleys to use to suit their needs, whereas Charlotte's limited choice of trolley can actually prevent her from being able to do her shopping. Even if an average-sized person only needed to pick up a few items, they could still use a bigger trolley if no others were available. However, Charlotte's choice is limited, which means that her access to a more suitable trolley is dependent on how busy a supermarket is. Other participants also spoke about not being able to use a deep trolley which limits their choice of trolley and restricts their ability to shop. Two participants spoke about an alternative way of using a deep trolley when there are no shallow trolleys available:

Joan and Steve: *… If we can we get the shallow ones [trolleys]. If we have to use a deep one, we put a couple of the handbaskets in it so that I can reach in and just pull the basket out.*

The alternative of placing handbaskets in a deep trolley allows Joan and Steve to still be able to use a deep trolley when the shallow ones are not available, increasing their choice of trolley. The handbaskets reduce how far they have to reach inside the trolley, and thus Joan and Steve show resistance to an otherwise disabling situation. Joan is 4' 2" and Steve is 4' 6" (making Steve the tallest participant and Joan above average). This may be why they are able to use a deep trolley and still reach the handbaskets within them. Other people with dwarfism who are below the average stature for someone with the impairment may not be able to use this alternative. Joan and Steve also point out the problems of using a trolley due to the height of the handlebar:

Steve: *You've [to Joan] nearly lost your teeth a couple of times [laughs]. If someone bangs into you, the trolley hits your mouth.*

Joan: *They have got new trolleys now with a little clipboard thing where you can put your shopping list, and they sort of take my view.*

Even when they can use a trolley, it can still present difficulties, including injury. The handlebar is likely to be face level to some with dwarfism, meaning that it will be difficult to see over. The accessory placed on the handlebar is another addition which aids people when shopping, but causes a hindrance for people with dwarfism. The lack of suitable trolleys and additional assistance for other shoppers all contribute to telling people with dwarfism that they are out of place. They are out of place in the sense that their needs are not catered to whilst the needs of other shoppers are. The additional accessories are used to entice customers to use their supermarket in order to increase profits rather than supermarkets catering to the needs of their shoppers. This demonstrates that no consideration is given to their disabling consequences for people with dwarfism who due to their small numbers are unlikely to affect a supermarket's profits if they were to stop shopping there. A lack of access can lead to people with dwarfism avoiding certain spaces.

Due to the number of difficulties when shopping, three participants mentioned how they have now begun to do their shopping online. As of January 2019, it is estimated that in the UK, 20% of shopping was done online (Office of National Statistics, 2019). Most of the big supermarket retailers in the UK now offer their services online and provide door-to-door deliveries at an extra cost. Online shopping means that people with dwarfism can avoid the numerous socio-spatial barriers mentioned previously:

Lydia: *My only difficulty I would find is packing my bags and possibly reaching the payment system because sometimes they have them out on an arm and you can't always reach them. I hate big, deep trolleys. I do my entire supermarket shopping online now… It is just so much easier to get someone else to do it for you.*

Michelle: *I don't really like shopping, we do it online shopping. If I can't get it done online, I take my son with me because he helps a lot. Our local Asda [British supermarket owned by Walmart] has even made the height of their trolleys even higher now than what they used to be. I only noticed that a few weeks ago. I try to do a big online shop and then if I need anything else, I use the smaller trolley.*

For Michelle, her average-sized son can help with shopping, but of course this will be dependent on his availability. Whilst Michelle can receive assistance from her son, this may not be possible for other people with dwarfism who may live alone. Online shopping allows people with dwarfism to shop from the comfort of their own homes at any time. It is a form of shopping that is dependent on an average-sized worker to shop and deliver groceries to them, removing all disabling barriers. It is a useful form of shopping, but it highlights how inaccessible typical supermarkets are and how they restrict their access to other members of the public. For Jade this makes her feel isolated and not part of the community:

Jade: *I used to get assistance with shopping through social services, but now I don't because of cuts. They [Social services] think I can manage it on my own, and yet the shopping trolley is bigger than me. So they told me to do online shopping, so you don't get out and get the chance to meet people. You don't get to be part of the community, you become isolated.*

Jade had to begin doing her shopping online due to economic cuts and a presumption by social services professionals, who are meant to help remove disabling barriers experienced by people with impairments, that she was capable of doing her shopping by herself. Shakespeare et al. (2007) suggest that other members of the public make assumptions about the abilities of people with dwarfism, which are often inaccurate. In this case, social services presumed Jade did not need any assistance despite the number of disabling barriers she encounters when shopping. Online shopping should be a *choice* for people with dwarfism, in the same way that it is for the average-sized person. Providing facilities that are more appropriate or assistance when shopping would mean that online shopping would become a *choice* for people with dwarfism. However, to get to these spaces, there must also be an accessible form of transport available.

2.3.1 (In)accessible transport

Accessible public transport is key in ensuring that disabled people can commute between different spaces, including for leisure, social and employment purposes. However, public transport has been shown to be inaccessible for disabled people (Gilderbloom and Rosentraub, 1990; Hine, 2016; Imrie, 1996; Øksenholt and Aarhaug, 2018). Gilderbloom and Rosentraub (1990) argue that public spaces become an 'invisible jail' for disabled people when public transport is unsuitable for them. They become confined to limited spaces. This prevents them from full access to public spaces and, in some cases, restrictions in accessing social events. According to Hine (2016: 21) 'differential levels of access to modes of transport (transport disadvantage) are also linked to social exclusion and poor access to goods and services'. It is not enough to make spaces and facilities that are in situ, such as buildings, accessible; these spaces must also be accessible through the use of different transport systems. Although many changes have been made to public transport to make it more accessible, such as automatic doors on trains and low-level buses, public transport still contains various socio-spatial barriers which cause access problems.

If public transport is not fully accessible, this can inhibit access to particular spaces for people with dwarfism. In terms of public transport, a number of participants mentioned various socio-spatial barriers, which caused difficulties, including when travelling by train:

Ivy: *I am not very good at getting up the steps on trains.*
Monica: *Trains are really difficult to get on.*

Several participants mentioned that the large gap between the train and the platform made it difficult for them to embark and disembark a train. Like with other forms of public transport trains, run by a strict time schedule and thus people are expected to board and disembark in a manner which matches the time schedule. If it takes longer to get on and off a train, this disrupts the normal time flow, which for Jade's case causes social problems:

Jade: *I really struggle because a lot of the trains and platforms don't match so there is a big step... people are so concerned with getting on the train at busy times they will push past you.*

It is not to be ignored that most commuters will encounter people pushing and shoving when getting on or off a train, especially during rush hour, but Jade's small stature places her in a more vulnerable situation than other commuters. Getting off trains also proved difficult, especially on older trains, as not only is there a large gap between the train and the platform, but also because many older trains do not have automatic doors:

Charlotte: *The only thing I do have problems with is with some old trains when you have to open the window to open the door. I panic if the train is empty as I need somebody to open the door for me. It's not so bad no though as most trains have automatic doors.*
Monica: *I can remember on the old trains and you had to stick your arm out of the window to open the door and I could never reach. It is always about having to problem solve and be one step ahead. If you are sitting on a train and it is late at night and you are the only one on a carriage [stop], I remember walking through carriages to try and find somebody who could open the door so that I didn't get stuck on the train.*

As Monica points out, encountering a socio-spatial barrier involves the extra labour of having to think ahead and to find someone to help her as opposed to being able to deal with a supposedly straightforward task. Of course, trains are busier at certain times, and thus Monica is likely to be more anxious about finding help late at night and thus will have to work harder to find assistance. When participants spoke about the older trains being difficult to open, they often spoke in the past tense. Older trains are now being phased out and newer trains are equipped with electronic buttons to open the doors, making them more accessible to a wider range of people, including people with dwarfism. These lower level buttons are a result of the Disability Discrimination Act (1995), which requires access to be provided where reasonable. However, it seems that not all train companies provide this reasonable access as it can be argued that many disabled people, particularly wheelchair users, require assistance when travelling by train and thus can rely on someone else to open the doors. It is only by ensuring that the button is low enough that it will still be accessible, as Amanda explains:

Amanda: *I will sometimes use the train but, I find with some trains the buttons to open the doors to get from one carriage to another can sometimes be too high. It depends on what train you get on but you can't always be sure that the train will be ok.*

It is not possible to determine whether or not the train Amanda needs to get on will be accessible, and therefore it is only when Amanda is on the train that she will find out whether she will encounter a disabling situation. This is problematic because once Amanda is on the train she is left with that barrier for the duration of her journey. The lack of consistency in regards to accessibility leaves people with dwarfism in unpredictable situations. Another problem, as Joan and Steve point out, is getting on the seat when travelling by coach and this again is dependent on whether an accessible coach is available:

Joan and Steve: *My problem often with coaches is the actual seat, getting in… If there is a solid arm, I can't get on. In some coaches before you get to the seat there is another step so they are very high. I have got to get onto the step before I can get on to the seat. If we have to go on a coach trip, we ask for the long seat at the back because it is easier to get on those.*

Joan and Steve demonstrate that their choice of seating is restricted. Seating is made to a specific standard, which can be disabling for people whose body size exceeds the norm. They become restricted in their choice of seating, which could be problematic if it is not vacant. Huff (2009) explores how seating is made to fit the average-sized person, and people who do not fit these standards are required to change in order to fit specific standards set out by corporations as opposed to these spaces being adapted to suit a range of individuals. Drawing on mass production as an example, Huff (2009) claims that creating products to a specific standard of size increases profits for corporations whilst relying on the user to adapt their body size. As Huff (2009) points out, the introduction of paying for two seats by some airlines shows that the blame is placed on the person as opposed to the airlines failing to provide for needs of the general population. Whilst Joan and Steve can possibly use the seating at the back of the bus, it still demonstrates how seating is restrictive to a wide range of people. Public transport services provide limited seating, but to further increase profits also sell more tickets than seats available. As a result, many passengers have to stand when travelling. This is problematic for people with dwarfism. First, people with dwarfism will not be able to reach some of the rails provided to other passengers to hold onto when standing. For example, many buses have hand rails that hang from the ceiling, which are obviously out of reach for people with dwarfism. Second, if the bus is crowded, they will be knocked and shoved by other passengers who are bigger than them. Last, as pointed out, people with dwarfism often have mobility impairment, which can make standing difficult. To overcome this problem for disabled passengers, busses and trains in the UK usually have reserved seats for disabled passengers, as indicated by the signs next to them. Non-disabled passengers are expected to give up these seats for disabled users. Some participants pointed out that there is still no guarantee of getting a seat, due to perception of disability and dwarfism:

Erin: *Do you find it difficult to get a seat [on public transport]?*
Tracy: *People, they look at you and think you are alright. I try not to go at busy times…. The other problem is standing up. Trains seem busier now. I don't cope well with standing up for long periods and, if you can't pre-book your ticket or if you do pre-book your ticket but the trains cancel that or if there is somebody in your seat, the general public do not see short people as being disabled.*

As Tracy points out, other members of the public do not recognise their difficulties, such as not being able to stand for long periods of time. For Tracy this affects when she travels, avoiding busy times. To overcome the problem of standing or using a seat that is unsuitable for her, Jade sits on her own suitcase:

Jade: *What I tend to do on a long journey and if it is busy, I will sit on my own suitcase. It's more comfortable.*

Sitting on her suitcase provides a way for Jade to have her own seat without having to ask anyone to give up theirs; people may be reluctant as they may not see her in need of a seat. As Jade points out, the seats are not suitable for her body size. Hettrick and Attig (2009) point out how seating, with reference to fat people, is unsuitable for their body size resulting in discomfort. Similarly, seating can also be uncomfortable for people with dwarfism:

Lydia: *I do find airplanes uncomfortable purely because of the ergonomics of the seating, and certain train seats are uncomfortable. One size fits all, and it doesn't fit all sizes does it? On a long journey on a plane or a train can be uncomfortable.*

This quote relates to spaces only being designed for particular bodily standards that lead to uncomfortable seating. It can be argued that a variety of passengers find seating on airplanes uncomfortable for other reasons, such as a lack of legroom. Whilst people often assume that people with dwarfism benefit from extra leg room on public transport, in reality, they encounter a number of difficulties. Monica also points out the problems of using busses and their seats being difficult for people with dwarfism to use:

Monica: *Busses are easier to get on now because they are lower, but we still can't very often reach the ticket machine and also sitting on a bus when it is going around corners can be scary because our feet don't reach the floor. We can be thrown all over the place.*

New busses are now partially accessible because their floors can be lowered to allow a wheelchair user access, which of course is also more appropriate for people with dwarfism as it makes getting on the bus easier if the distance from the pavement to the bus door is smaller. Despite this, due to other socio-spatial barriers, buses are not fully accessible. Again, Monica shows that the seating is part of the problem but this time it can also pose a safety risk. Most participants spoke about avoiding using busses for a number of reasons, including the busses stopping too far from their destination which is especially problematic for those with a mobility impairment. Arial mentions that the difficulties of using public transport limit how often she travels:

Erin: *Do you drive?*
Arial: *No, and I would like to because I could go to more places including more events [held by associations for people with dwarfism]. I only go to some, the ones which are held over a weekend, because travelling by public transport is so difficult.*

Arial is a widow and spoke about past experiences when her husband would drive them both to different places, thus avoiding public transport. Using public transport to only travel to events that are held over longer periods of time, such as over a weekend as opposed to a one-day event, suggests that the benefits of the event outweigh the cons of public transport. Barnes (1991a) suggests that transport that is not fully accessible restricts disabled people's access to social and leisure activities. This can include events held by associations for people with dwarfism that hold both leisure activities and the chance to socialise with others. Due to the many socio-spatial encounters people with dwarfism experience when using public transport, several spoke about how they preferred driving their own car. A car that has been modified to suit their body size, such as pedal extensions, is an ideal mode of transportation. However, such modifications can be expensive and are not necessarily covered by any government grants for disability accommodations. Despite this, Amanda points out why she prefers using the car over public transport:

Amanda: *I don't really use public transport. I drive to most places. I will*
            sometimes use the train, but I find if I have to make a connection I
            can't always make it to the other train on time and have to wait a
            long time for another.

Missing her connection results in Amanda taking even longer to complete a
journey, demonstrating two forms of time disadvantage. First, she is at a
disadvantage as the connection time between trains only accounts for faster
walkers than her. Second, missing her original connection can add extra time
to her journey. Again, this is where a train's time schedule is inappropriate for
someone who takes longer to do something. Driving a car places her at the
same advantage as any other road user. Being able to drive a car, Kruse
(2003) points out, rids people with dwarfism of both social restraints and
socio-spatial barriers as they also provide anonymity from other members of
the public from whom they may receive unwanted attention. It is only when
having to refuel that socio-spatial barriers are encountered due to the way
some petrol stations have been designed and constructed as Amanda and
Amy point out:

Amy: *... the only thing about driving that is starting to get me at the*
            moment is the petrol pumps in garages ... the pumps seem to be
            higher. When they are putting the new ones in, because they are
            putting longer tubes in so that they are not missing people who
            can't get the pump in the right side who would just drive off to the
            next garage, they have now put longer tubes on so that they can
            reach round and fill the other side of their car up. This of course
            means that they have got to put the pumps up higher.
Amanda: *... some garages have put on their pumps a choice for you to pay at*
            the pump or in the kiosk. You have to put in your choice first before
            filling your car but I can't reach so I can't use any garage which
            has that system.

Amy is a mother of two children, one of whom has cerebral palsy, and she
relies on driving a van in order to take her son to and from hospital in
London. Although she spoke about the van being easier to use than public
transport, she is still met with socio-spatial barriers when driving. Across the
UK, many petrol stations are introducing new pumps that aim to provide
more choice to the average consumer. These petrol stations are only considering the needs of the average-sized user, rendering disabled people out of
place in more ways than one. These choices are aimed at encouraging more
drivers to use their petrol stations and thus increasing the company's profits.
Thus, the facilities are implemented with economic advantages in mind as
opposed to the range of customers and their different needs. Again, this
relates to putting the needs of corporations before the various customers.
Creating an average customer means producing facilities that are also all the

same. Huff (2009) argues that the mass production of facilities provides high profit margins through the production of quick and cheap products. It can be argued that this approach to customer choice for average-sized people actually takes away Amy and Amanda's ability to even refuel their car let alone decide on where they want to pay or which pump they want to use.

One way of overcoming the problems often faced within a petrol station is by having an attendant refuelling a person's car. In some UK garages, attendants are readily available, but in other cases assistance from an attendant is only available if a person has a blue badge, as Joanne points out:

Joanne: *Another situation that is a real challenge for me as a dwarf is the petrol station. This is where the blue badge[1] is a godsend. I put the badge up on my dashboard to notify the people in the kiosk that I am a disabled person.*

A blue badge provides disabled people with certain exemptions when driving, in this case, the opportunity for assistance when refuelling. As not all participants considered themselves to be disabled, they may not all have a blue badge, or they may not have qualified for a blue badge due to restrictions within the scheme. Thus, this assistance will not be available to all of them, leaving them still encountering difficulties when at the petrol station. In their report on living with dwarfism in the UK, Shakespeare et al. (2007) found that just over half of their participants had a blue badge, despite recognising a number of benefits it would give (Chapter 4, *Disabling identities*, will discuss in more detail how people's perceptions of disability can affect people with dwarfism receiving assistance and access to accessible spaces). Despite the assistance being available at a petrol station, Sofia points out how it can be difficult accessing disability assistance:

Sofia: *It's like at Asda [British supermarket] at their petrol station you need to press a button to ring for attention to help fill up but is really high up and even someone in a wheelchair would have trouble reaching.*

The inaccessibility of the facility suggests that there is a lack of consideration given as to how public spaces contribute to a person's disablement. More thought needs to be given when implementing facilities. It seems that there is a lack of thought being given to a disabled person's needs. This calls into question to what degree spaces labelled as "accessible" are truly accessible.

This section has shown how everyday spaces and facilities are usually inaccessible and in some cases impossible for people with dwarfism to access. People with dwarfism often have difficulties in using facilities that are easily accessible to the general public (Shakespeare et al., 2007). These socio-spatial barriers to inclusion are clearly evident in public spaces, for example chip and pin machines being placed too high and out of reach for people with dwarfism. As Wendell (1996) suggests, buildings and objects cause disability as they are created for too narrow a range of people. People with dwarfism would encounter fewer disabling situations if they were accessible for a more diverse range of users.

In a number of cases, participants encountered socio-spatial barriers when a facility had been altered in order to increase economic opportunities for companies by providing increased choice to non-disabled users. Oliver (1990) contends new technologies should be used to liberate disabled people as opposed to further disabling them. Increasing the economic advantages for companies not only infringes on a person's right to access spaces and facilities but also demonstrates that no thought has been put into providing access for them; this further tells them that they do not belong. These facilities are relatively new, for example, self-service checkouts were first used in UK supermarkets in 2002, thus it can be suggested that some spaces are becoming more disabling as opposed to enabling for a wide range of users. This contradicts the UK's supposedly offering access for disabled people, evident in legislation such as the Equality Act (2010). Whilst there are accessible facilities and spaces (which will be discussed in the next section), other spaces are becoming more disabling thereby limiting the rights of people with dwarfism.

This section has shown that public spaces create many disabling experiences for people with dwarfism and the different ways they resist socio-spatial barriers. For disabled people, public transport results in constraints and compromise (Porter, 2000). In a number of cases, participants had to make compromises in order to be able to access public transport, such as only sitting in particular spaces. They also encountered constraints, such as lack of choice of petrol station and pursuing leisure activities. The disabling encounters for people with dwarfism need to be made more apparent in society. As physical barriers within public spaces are a contributing factor to a person's disablement, modifications to public spaces can also make them enabling (Imrie, 1996b). The next section explores whether accessible spaces provide people with dwarfism with greater access to public spaces.

2.4 (In)Accessible spaces

In order to create a broader understanding of disablement, it is relevant to explore how people with dwarfism interact with supposedly accessible spaces, also more commonly known as 'disabled spaces'. Due to the realisation that public spaces can be disabling for people with impairments, spaces are now being adapted in order to provide access. Also known as accessible spaces, accessible spaces are a response to an inaccessible built environment. Hahn (1986) argues that accessible environments are possible through changing the laws and policies that exist. In the UK there are numerous disability access polices, such as Part M of the Buildings and Regulations Act (2010). The main aim is to provide reasonable accommodations that adhere to the Disability Discrimination Act (1995), which has since been replaced by the Equality Act (2010). As well as in the UK, there are also other numerous policies and legislation, such as the Americans with Disabilities Act (1990), the Australian Disability Discrimination Act 1992, Accessible Canada Bill (2019) and many others. The UN convention on the Rights of Persons with Disabilities also stresses that disabled people should have access to transport and the built environment. The convention has been signed by 162 countries.

Whilst there are laws and policies pertaining to disability access, how each country perceives disability can impact who is provided with appropriate access. Within the UK, there are spaces that aim to provide better access to spaces for disabled people, including tactile paving for people with visual impairments and drop kerbs for wheelchair users, which should provide increased access for disabled people. In this section, I question whether 'accessible' spaces actually help to reduce disablement for people with dwarfism or if they are just another spatial barrier. Hahn (1986) suggests that public policies reflect prevalent social attitudes and values towards disabled people. Different researchers have engaged with how policies affect the implementation of accessible spaces (Barnes, 1991a; Hahn, 1986; Imrie and Kumar, 1998; Imrie and Wells, 1993). Imrie and Kumar (1998) suggest that access for disabled people is done to a bare minimum, as it is seen as the exception rather than the rule. This bare minimum often reflects a problematic construction of disability, which does not include body sizes that exceed the norm. In the UK, laws and policies relating to disability access often have a narrow view of what disability is, and thus access is usually only provided for a narrow range of disabled people. For example, in Part M of the Buildings and Regulations Act (2010), 'Access to and use of Buildings: Volume 2 – Buildings other than Dwellings', attention to access is biased towards wheelchair users. In only two parts of the Act are people with dwarfism included. In Part M, people with dwarfism are offered a second handrail and access to lower ticket machines. However, all other lower facilities are deemed to be reachable by wheelchair users. This is problematic for people with dwarfism who are shorter than the average wheelchair user. The average stature of a wheelchair user is considered to be 4' 6" (137 cm), whereas the average stature of a person with dwarfism is 4' (122 cm). This makes them significantly shorter and, added to this, most people with dwarfism are unable to reach over their head. It is presumed that a wheelchair user has an average arm reach.

Chouinard (1999b) explores the importance of recognising disabled people, not as a homogenous group, but as a group made up of people with various impairments, which are not always obvious within society. Although disabled people share common experiences, it still needs to be recognised that the experiences of different impairment groups vary (Shakespeare et al., 2010). This becomes problematic if planners are to create an "accessible" space with only a particular group of impairments in mind. I argue that because dwarfism is not a common impairment and often its identity as a disability is contested, then implementing accessible spaces suitable for them will be minimal, or ignored. Despite this, it can be argued that some accessible spaces do provide better access as Myraar and Naomi state:

Myraar: *I think in banks they have a lower desk which is quite good and at the GPs they are lower ... I go to the lower desk and wait for them to come and help. I have tried to go to the upper desk and they can't see me, so I always use the lower desk.*

Naomi: *I think a lot of disabled facilities have improved now. I can use cash machines which were lowered for disabled people. Now that everything has got to be DDA [Disability Discrimination Act 1995] compliant, everything has to be wheelchair level which is also my level.*

In various spaces, low counters have been installed in order to comply with disability legislation, including the Disability Discrimination Act (1995) and Equality Act (2010), which remove an otherwise disabling situation. Although the facilities may have been lowered for wheelchair users, the coincidence in height also allows Myraar and Naomi better access. Low-level counters are between 750 and 800 mm, just less than three feet from the floor (Good Access Guide, 2002). The average height for a standard counter is between 1000 and 1200 mm, which is between three feet, three inches and just under four feet (ibid). Heights of the participants ranged from 3' 2" to 4' 6", although most participants were less than four feet tall. The height of the participants and the height of a standard counter would mean that most of them would barely be able to see over a standard counter, and, due to their short arm length, they would also have difficulty reaching across the counter, such as in order to pass or sign documents. This demonstrates that, for participants, the standard counters would either be difficult or impossible to use. Although some places do provide low counters, using them is not always possible for a number of reasons which Ivy and Joanne talk about:

Ivy: *I was admitted to hospital a few years back, and, when we went up to the counter to register, the lady on the desk, I could barely see her, and I didn't know at that time that there was a lower desk but it was all cluttered up with files. This lady asked me for my name, and I said my name, and she said the name of somebody else, and I said she looked at my husband and said, 'you will have to speak for her. I can't hear her and I can't see her'.*

Joanne: *I've found recently that pharmacies and new build doctors surgeries have really high reception desks. I'm really frustrated with their reception area which is enclosed behind glass panes ... they have trouble hearing me as I position myself at the lower end of the desk furthest away from them so I can actually see them comfortably.*

Frustratingly, the lower part of the desk the glass panes are covered in surgery notices which makes it even more awkward for me to talk to the receptionist. There seems to have been no thought process here ... either that or there is real lack of disabled access awareness on part of the staff. You can gain access into the buildings ok, but trying to access the service at the first hurdle at the reception presents a barrier and is not particularly welcoming for people with disabilities.

The member of staff communicated with Ivy's husband, who is of average stature, despite the fact that it was Ivy's issue that they were dealing with and thus Ivy was made to feel out of place. These accessible spaces are still controlled by non-disabled people, who dominate public spaces, reflecting ableist values. Imrie (1996b) points out that accessible spaces are often misused. This demonstrates that providing access for disabled people, through changing the representation of the space is not enough. The misuse of these spaces reflects disablist practices that tell disabled people that they do not belong. An accessible space is made inaccessible by ableist attitudes that deem the average-sized person's needs, in this case the need to advertise surgery notices or to store files. The lack of consideration given suggests that there is little thought for disabled people and indicates that they do not belong in that space. Under the Equality Act (2010), members of staff who interact with members of the public are required to undertake disability awareness training (Directgov online, 2012). If the staff had dealt with the situations better, through better disability awareness, including keeping the low area of the desk clear and clutter free, the situations could have been avoided. Therefore, it shows that for a place to be fully accessible it is not enough to change the actual physical space but also the attitudes of people who manage those spaces.

Although a low counter provides better access, when it is not being misused, the way it has been designed and for whom can still cause some access issues. Monica suggests that although someone in a wheelchair is sitting down the assumption is that person still has an average reach:

Monica: ... *Apart from smaller counters and things, but even then people in wheelchairs have still got the reach as they have average-sized arms, whereas they don't think about it for us at all.*

The assumption is that all wheelchair users will have an average arm length unlike a person with dwarfism. Although Monica thinks no consideration has been given to people with dwarfism, this assumption can be broadened to include any impairment where a person has no arms or limited use of their arms. Chouinard (1999b) argues that 'accessible' spaces which do not adequately accommodate various impairments, result in disabled people still struggling for better physical access. This indicates that accessible spaces are based on the premise of a normalcy of disability, in other words the average disabled person. Only creating for this average disabled person is deemed more cost effective, but does not solve the problem of providing access for all. Only providing for a narrow range of people with impairments can leave people with dwarfism having to negotiate between accessible and non-accessible spaces.

Another accessible space which can be beneficial for people with dwarfism, provided it is designed appropriately, is a ramp. Only a few participants spoke about using a ramp but the ones who did found it to be usually easier to navigate than steps:

Joan and Steve: *If we are going into a building and there is a ramp or steps, we'll use the ramp... Steps do vary in depth. People don't understand, although you will understand, but a step is often the same height as our knee. If an average person went up steps as high as their knees, they would know... Also, the ramp is sometimes a lot longer. If there is only one or two steps then we will use the steps, if they are not very high steps.*

Kayleigh: *Steep steps I hate, but if you are doing the proper standard gradient of steps then I am fine.*

The representation of each space is based on a specific user and neither include a person with dwarfism. The lack of inclusion of people with dwarfism results in them having to negotiate a most suitable way of access. Despite the fact that ramps are mainly to provide access for wheelchair users, they can also be beneficial for people with dwarfism, due to some steps being too steep. All people with dwarfism have a shorter leg length than the average-sized person. However, a person with disproportionate dwarfism, such as Achondroplasia, is likely to have even shorter legs, resulting in more difficulty trying to climb a set of steps. Although Joan and Steve point out that if the ramp is very long and there are only one or two steps then they will use the steps instead, but only if they are not very high steps, showing that they have to assess the best means of access before entering a building. This is because having to walk up a long ramp takes longer and could be affected by their mobility difficulties, which they both spoke about, or steps may be too steep and difficult to get up due to their body size. The use of ramps and steps, depending on their construction, demonstrates a multitude of different ways of accessing or not being able to access a space.

Another accessible space that people with dwarfism have to assess in terms of access is the accessible toilet. An accessible toilet should provide direct access, however, the materiality of the space can be difficult to negotiate due to for whom it has been constructed. Kitchin and Law (2001) examine how public toilets in Ireland are often poorly designed and do not adequately provide access for disabled people. The research consisted of interviews with disabled people, many of whom were wheelchair users, and an examination of planning legislation in the UK. Their study points out that not providing adequate accessible toilets is an infringement on the rights of disabled people. What was also interesting in their study was that public toilets, which were meant to be accessible for disabled people, were often inaccessible and showed that the different needs of disabled people were not taken into account. This lack of full accessibility is also apparent for people with dwarfism:

Lydia: *Disabled toilets are often, the actual toilet which is porcelain is very often high, but it is high because they are assuming that the disabled person is a wheelchair user and needs it that high to transfer from wheelchair to toilet so often it is too high for us to get onto.*

Jade: *The toilets that say they are for disabled people have got really high seats so you have to climb on them. The good thing about them is that you can reach the sink and you can see the mirror and you can lock the door safely.*

A partially accessible toilet leaves people with dwarfism in a catch-22 situation. They can either struggle to get onto the accessible toilet and then be able to use the lower facilities, or they can use a non-disabled toilet and struggle to use the other facilities, such as the sink. Accessible spaces do not accommodate for all impairments and in some cases can cause further difficulties for them (Chouinard, 1999a). Despite being disabled, they are still made to feel out of place within a space designed to provide access for disabled people. Kitchin and Law (2001) argue that the socio-spatial construction of accessible toilets makes them unsuitable for a range of disabled people as they are often built with a very narrow view of how they will be used and by whom. The conception of an accessible toilet is that it is to provide access for disabled people, however, these spaces are only constructed with a narrow conception of disabled people, which does not encompass people with dwarfism. According to Lefebvre (1991), a space is a social product that is produced through perceptions of the body. How the disabled body is perceived within society will result in accessible spaces reflecting that identity. As disability is perceived as a mobility impairment, signified by the use of a wheelchair, then an accessible space will be constructed with that user in mind. The access needs of people with dwarfism differ from wheelchair users, resulting in people with dwarfism having to assess how accessible an accessible space actually is.

Due to accessible toilets not being fully accessible because of the height of the actual toilet, three participants mentioned carrying their own hand sanitisers with them. This was so that they could use the non-disabled toilets whilst avoiding some of the inaccessible facilities, as Naomi points out:

Naomi: *I don't use a disabled toilet. I use a normal toilet. The sinks are a bit of a pain, but the biggest problem is the soap, so I carry wet wipes with me.*

Although it is not uncommon to see people using their own hand sanitisers in public toilets, Naomi having to use her own because she cannot reach the soap dispenser, which tends to be placed high up on a wall above the sinks, shows that she does not have the same level of access as other people. Using their own hand sanitiser indicates that some of the participants have to provide their own form of adaptation which shows resistance and agency to an otherwise disabling situation.

2.4.1 (In)Accessible spaces—a hierarchy of impairments

It can be argued that if accessible spaces do not accommodate for people with dwarfism then they are another exclusionary space. Accessible spaces for people with physical impairments often meet the needs of only certain impairments, leaving others to be ignored (Bickenbach et al., 1999). Over half of the participants believed that accessible spaces helped to make them feel more included within public spaces. What made them feel excluded was when accessible spaces where designed to solely benefit wheelchair users as Amanda and Sofia explain:

Erin: *Do these facilities help you to feel included within everyday society or excluded?*

Amanda: *I suppose excluded because, although it's good to have some things at your height, you know they haven't done it for you, it's for a wheelchair user, and so your needs haven't been taken into account. I think planners should be more open-minded when it comes to disability and think that it is not just people in wheelchairs that need help.*

Sofia: *Here in England they only see disabled people as people in wheelchairs. I do feel we are excluded and not seen as important as other disabled people.*

Although both Amanda and Sofia recognised themselves as disabled, they feel excluded by the unsuitable facilities and not seen as just as important as people with other impairments. Positive changes have been made within public spaces, such as the implementation of ramps and drop kerbs, but these facilities have been implemented with the aim of providing access for mostly wheelchair users, and to Sofia this shows they are thought of as more important, creating a hierarchy of impairments. Imrie (2012) comments that design solutions for disabled people often revolve around the provision of wheelchair access and do not cater for a wider range of disabled people. This may be because it is seen as more beneficial and economical to provide for a more common impairment as opposed to an impairment such as dwarfism.

Despite not providing full access, accessible spaces do help to provide some access and thus, as Grace points out, makes her feel included:

Erin: *Do these facilities help you to feel included within everyday society or excluded?*

Grace: *Definitely included as light switches and other things are usually lower and it changes so much for you. Other people can also use them as they are not too low, but it means you are more independent and included, there should be more compromises like that.*

Grace is given more independence and one less socio-spatial barrier to face when out in public simply if a facility is lowered. This shows that if accessible spaces were designed and implemented to suit a wider range of people, then people with dwarfism can feel more included within society. Despite this, Myraar points out that how people respond to her using accessible spaces can make her feel excluded:

Erin: *Do you think disabled facilities help you to feel more included within everyday society?*

Myraar: *Yes, but I think you feel quite different when you are using some things like lower cash machines as people are staring at you, and then you feel that it is made just for you. As long as you access it then it is ok.*

Erin: *So, the facility makes you feel included but the way people act towards you using it doesn't?*

Myraar: *Yes.*

Myraar points out that accessible spaces do make public spaces feel more inclusive, but that unwanted social encounters are created when using them. Butler and Bowlby (1997) suggest that disabled people are often looked at and perceived as a social curiosity, and this is likely to affect their use of their bodies. It is not unusual for people with dwarfism to be stared at, however, using an accessible space may prompt other people to stare as they are likely to be intrigued as to how they manage different spaces. What can encourage this behaviour is the representation of the accessible space. Accessible spaces are often segregated from their non-disabled counterparts (Imrie, 1996b). This can indicate that disabled people are different. Kitchin (1998) suggests that accessible spaces often show disabled people as different and out of place. Naomi backs up Myraar's claim and suggests that to feel included is to have accessible which blend in with the rest of the place:

Naomi: *I think the best disabled facilities are the ones nobody else notices, like lift buttons, low cash machines and low light switches. I think things like bubbly paving at crossings which are now seen as indications to everyone as a place to cross. It's handy for visually impaired people but it's also just a part of the street. It's not seen as abnormal. It's the same with dropped kerbs, which not only benefits disabled people but also people with pushchairs and bicycles.*

For Naomi, who mentioned a lot in her interview about receiving unwanted attention, in order for a disabled facility or space to be inclusive, they have to be well designed and unnoticeable. Making a space which blends in with the rest of the built environment and being usable by a range of different users makes it more inclusive and helps to rid the notion of disabled people as different and 'out of place'. This could be done by ensuring accessible places are not located in different spaces to regular facilities, such as back door access or segregated accessible toilets, but instead by designing and constructing the built environment for a greater diversity of users from the start.

This section has shown that accessible spaces can be enabling and disabling for people with dwarfism, depending on how the space has been constructed and who for. Whilst participants felt that accessible spaces are mainly designed and implemented with wheelchair users in mind, these spaces can be beneficial for them, especially if they have been lowered. This can often help to remove a socio-spatial barrier, giving people with dwarfism access to more spaces. Despite this, Shakespeare (2006) points out that accessible spaces can cause conflict between people with different impairments, as providing for one impairments group can cause disablement for another. A prime example of this was shown when participants spoke about the height of the toilet in the accessible spaces being too high as it is designed for a wheelchair user's needs.

Only certain impairments are considered within 'accessible' public spaces, through the design of spaces suitable for their needs. The needs of people with dwarfism are often met through the coincidence of some of their needs matching that of a wheelchair user, such as lower facilities. Planners and local authorities are often biased towards catering for wheelchair users when implementing disabled facilities (Imrie and Kumar, 1998). This is not to ignore that these facilities are beneficial, not only for wheelchair users but to increase their effectiveness then more impairments need to be accounted for. As Hahn (1986) states, planners need to be aware of the many people with impairments who do not necessarily use a wheelchair. If the accessible spaces were designed for a range of users, then they would be more beneficial to a greater number of users. Taking into account a broader range of impairments and designing public spaces for this reason can help to overcome a larger range of socio-spatial barriers for disabled people.

There is a normalcy of disability which affects the provision of inclusive design being fully accessible for people with dwarfism. Disability access is partly reflective of capitalist agendas to increase profits for corporations. Providing minimum access saves costs but does not provide full access for people with dwarfism. Disguising disability as something which is visible, or more specifically a wheelchair user, allows for minimal costs to be spent on access. This is enough to satisfy some disabled people and enough for non-disabled people to argue that enough has been done to provide access for all disabled people. Those of us who do not benefit from the supposed accessible spaces, in this case people with dwarfism, can be deemed unreasonable as they are expecting too much. The accommodations are an extra cost, and this is problematic when disabled people are already being deemed an economic burden.

2.5 Infantilising spaces

This last section of this chapter explores how spaces constructed for children can be enabling or disabling for people with dwarfism. This does not necessarily refer to playgrounds, but rather spaces that corporations have implemented either to prevent children accessing or to purposely increase children's access to them. As people with dwarfism and children are of similar stature, the purpose of the child facility or space can have the same effect on people with dwarfism. This, of course, depends on the purpose of the space. If it is thought that the space or facility may be misused by children then it will probably be put out of their reach. A space that is unsuitable for a child will not affect an adult of average stature, but will disable someone with dwarfism. On the other hand, if a space is created for children, it is likely to benefit people with dwarfism. Jennifer talks about how she is unable to use a facility, as she believes it has been purposely put out of place to prevent children from misusing it:

Jennifer: *A good example of that [a child barrier] is the meat ticket machine in the supermarket; you know where you get your number. I can only imagine that that is high up to stop every kid wanting to take a ticket. On the other hand, my solution to that is to get somebody to get me a ticket.*

It is interesting to note that the reason why the facility is put out of place is to stop children misusing it. It can be contended that the way a child responds and behaves in a particular space is taken into account before the needs of someone with dwarfism. Accommodating for children before people with dwarfism may be because there are more children within society and thus adapting for them is more practical and economical. However, this infantilises people with dwarfism and leaves them dependent on others. Furthermore, having the same access as children can be problematic when working with children, Tracy points out:

Tracy: *I remember I did a childcare course and where I did some of my training, I used to think, how am I supposed to get through that door? The handle was out of reach. I know it's to stop the children getting out but there are supposed to be like equal opportunities, and they're not any sort of thing.*

Working with children will obviously result in having to interact with spaces specifically for them. This means that the representation of a space changes and has implications on the spatial practices of people with dwarfism who wish to work in these spaces. In this case, a door with a high handle on it to prevent children from getting out also has the same effect upon people with dwarfism. This puts both people with dwarfism and children in the same position. Bolt (2014) uses the term 'disablist infantilisation' to describe the way disabled people are often treated as children. To be treated like a child in society results in a lack of power and can construct the person as immature. This can be problematic when working with children, as it may impact upon how they perceive a person with dwarfism and subsequently how they treat them.

Although the reasons for constructing spaces for children may be valid, such as for safety reasons, it stills means that people with dwarfism are made to feel out of place. Similarly, Kayleigh sees particular child facilities as socio-spatial barriers that prevent her from accessing different spaces:

Kayleigh: *They are a huge barrier [child barriers]. Keypads and locks are always at a bad height. Getting into swimming pools at a hotel, and in Australia a lot of playgrounds have locks on them so, if I wanted to take my cousins to the playground, I find it really difficult… Sometimes I think it is necessary and sometimes I think it is overkill.*

The socio-spatial barriers that Kayleigh mentions have a lot to do with being able to access particular spaces that are associated with children, such as the playground. These barriers are reflective of ableism, which construe parents or guardians of children as average-sized adults, ignoring the fact that disabled people can be parents or guardians. There is a common belief that disabled people are asexual and thus cannot be parents, or more specifically that they are incapable of raising or looking after children (Olsen and Clarke, 2003). These problematic beliefs influence the representation of children's spaces. The number of disabling barriers associated with child space can have an adverse effect on parents with dwarfism and those who work with children:

Alison: *In the church that I go to, we have got a kitchen and obviously things like knives have to be put out of reach [of children], and it is not accessible at all for me. I find that very frustrating, and the storage cupboard that we have for the craft things is also really high up so that is frustrating.*

Alison mentioned in her interview that she helps out in her local church where she leads the children's club. The needs of both children and average-sized adults are considered before Alison's, resulting in an ableist situation.

Putting certain facilities out of reach of children prevents Alison from being able to carry out her duties as expected and forces her to be more reliant on the help of others.

Although there are some resources or equipment within child facilities and spaces which have been purposely put out of reach from children, there are some which have been lowered for the benefit of children. In some circumstances, providing resources that are accessible for children can also result in increased accessibility of public spaces for people with dwarfism:

Ivy: *I had a surprise one day when I went into the toilets in British Home Stores [British department store], and they had a low toilet there obviously for children, and I thought it was a good idea, and children would have a job reaching the taps and we encourage children to wash their hands.*

Lydia: *... In the Trafford centre [Out of town shopping centre in the north west of England] the toilets now not only do they have disabled toilets but they usually have the kid's area for young people and children. I would quite happily go and use the young people's sections because the sinks are lowered. Most of the time if you use the sink in the ladies toilets, you get wet armpits because you having to wash your hands above your shoulders and you get all the water running up your arms or the hand dryer is so far up you having to dry your hands above your head and you get all water trickling down you. It is whatever is suitable at the time...thay are more suitable for us as they are just the ame as the rest but lower.*

Children's toilets are implemented for somebody who is small in stature and thus are more suitable for people with dwarfism as the only adjustment made to all the facilities is a reduction in their height. A low sink allows people with dwarfism to wash their hands without struggling or having to take their own hand sanitisers. There is a parallel here with the arguments of Oliver (2004) who claims that implementing more accessible facilities to benefit some people in society can also benefit others. Ivy points out that the child toilets were a 'surprise' to her (indicating that she may have not come across this kind of facility before), they may not be available in a wide range of spaces. Unlike the (supposedly) accessible toilet, there is no legislation which makes it compulsory for such a space to exist. They are only implemented for economic purposes and thus are implemented to encourage parents to that particular space to spend money there. The economic reasoning for the space reflects Lefebvre (1991) argument that spaces are produced by capitalism. These spaces are only implemented to increase the economic opportunity of the space they are within, as opposed to providing access based on the needs of a wide range of users.

The probability of a person with dwarfism accessing a shopping centre is lower than the probability of a child accessing the same space. This means that it is more economical to provide an accessible space for children and thus the representation of the space will also reflect the needs of children. In other words, the space will be decorated with childish themes which indicate an infantilising space. Thus, whilst the materiality of the space is suitable for adults with dwarfism, the meaning of the space is not. Imrie (1996b) suggests that the built environment infantilises disabled people through paternalistic signs. I would like to add that child facilities that both enable and disable people with dwarfism also infantilise them as they place them in a similar situation to children (especially if other members of the public see them using them). Only children are expected to use these facilities, and thus an adult using them may be seen as childlike. In some cases, child spaces are segregated, emphasising their use for children and not adults. Providing spaces that are accessible for a wider range of people would remove infantilising situations.

Child facilities and spaces can both limit and increase access for people with dwarfism within public spaces, depending on the purpose of the facility or space. This comes down to similarities in body size between a child and a dwarf as facilities for a child are either lowered or placed out of reach of children depending on their purpose. Providing for the needs of children, whilst neglecting the access needs of people with dwarfism is another form of ableism that indicates to disabled people that they do not belong.

2.6 Conclusion

It is apparent that people with dwarfism encounter a number of socio-spatial barriers which are the result of a mismatch in height. This lack of access is based upon what body is perceived to be the productive occupant of that space (Lefebvre, 1991). This aligns with Longhurst's (2005, 2010) argument that the materiality of spaces can be disabling for people whose body size does not adhere to average standards. According to Lefebvre (1991) capitalism produces spaces. Spaces are mass-produced in order to benefit the norm, such as the average-sized, non-disabled person. Mass-producing spaces to accommodate for the majority is deemed less costly than producing spaces for a range of people. The drive to produce spaces for the average-sized person is becoming more problematic within neoliberal societies where businesses are constantly looking for ways to maximise profits.

Whilst in western societies there has been an increase in the implementation of accessible spaces, this has not necessarily produced a more accessible built environment as there has also been a drive to construct cost-effective spaces, which ignores the needs of disabled people. Furthermore, the construction of accessible spaces is also reflective of economic considerations, as they only accommodate for a narrow range of disabled people. In regards to accessible spaces, it is believed that a specific type of wheelchair user will be occupying that space. The rarity of dwarfism and its lack of recognition as a disability means that people with dwarfism are often not accommodated for. Accessible spaces are only partially accessible for people with dwarfism due to the coincidence of both them and wheelchair users requiring access to lower facilities.

The representation of spaces are produced by dominant ableist beliefs, which impact upon the spatial practices of people with dwarfism. People with dwarfism often have to find their own way of dealing with a socio-spatial barrier, which indicates that they do not belong. The adoption of disability access policies and legislation has not aided in providing full access for people with dwarfism. To create a truly inclusive built environment, the access needs to be for a range of people and needs to be considered and placed before profits.

Note

1 A Blue Badge is a parking permit awarded to disabled people who have mobility difficulties, providing them with exemptions in regards to parking, such as being permitted to park in accessible spaces and on double yellow lines. The blue badge in this case also notifies the garage that the person needs assistance when refuelling.

3 Resisting spaces

3.1 Introduction

The representation of a space changes the representational space for people with dwarfism, which as this chapter will show, impacts their spatial practices. Building on from the previous chapter, this chapter explores how people with dwarfism interact with socio-spatial barriers. First, people with dwarfism can avoid spaces which are inaccessible, thereby reducing the number of spaces. Psycho-emotional disablism involves the intended or unintended they access. Avoiding particular spaces because of inaccessibility means that disabled people will tend to confine their activities to places which are mostly barrier free (Hahn, 1986). Avoiding spaces means that people with dwarfism do not have the same equal access to the built environment as non-disabled people.

Second, to gain access and overcome socio-spatial barriers, people with dwarfism may employ their own management strategies, which will involve interacting with a space differently. Interacting with a space differently can involve either being dependent on someone else or can provoke different social interactions. This chapter explores the social interactions people with dwarfism encounter when they require assistance or do something differently. These interactions involve numerous management strategies.

First, this chapter engages with notions of dependency and disability, before exploring the literature focusing on the social interaction between disabled and non-disabled people. The chapter is then split into two analysis sections and lastly a conclusion. The first analysis section demonstrates some of the ways in which people with dwarfism negotiate socio-spatial barriers, through dependency and the resulting social interactions. Miller (1987) in Thompson, et al. (2008) suggests that, due to their small stature, people with dwarfism face socio-spatial barriers within public spaces which limit what they can do and therefore limits their independence. This section demonstrates how being dependent on someone else is not a straightforward task, but it is affected by social attitudes that are not always welcome. This section calls for more consideration of interdependence within society in order to normalise the extra degree of dependency people with dwarfism experience due to the built environment not being size suitable for them.

The second analysis section focuses on how people with dwarfism respond to different socio-spatial barriers in their own way, not only demonstrating some of the different management strategies they employ, but also exploring how other members of the public respond to their actions. This section focuses on issues of normalcy and how breaking from the norm provokes unwanted attention in particular spaces and situations. This section demonstrates how the attitudes and responses from other members of the public can be as disabling as the actual socio-spatial barrier.

3.2 Dependency and social interactions between disabled and non-disabled people

A number of researchers have explored notions of dependency in relation to disability (Kittay, 2011; Kittay, et al., 2005; Morris, 1991, 2001; Oliver, 1989, 1990; Rock, 1988). Dependency can be defined as 'the inability to do something for oneself and consequently the reliance upon others to carry out some or all of the tasks of everyday life' (Oliver, 1990: 83). For disabled people, dependency can either be the result of a functional limitation or because of the built environment. Spaces are purposely constructed to ensure that the average-sized, able-bodied person can interact with spaces independently. The way the built environment has been constructed affects the independence of people with impairments (Imrie and Hall, 2001).

On the other hand, independence, as we know it, has been claimed to be fictitious (Morris, 1991). Interdependency claims that everyone is dependent on each other. Within the built environment both disabled people and other members of the public are not completely independent in the sense that they rely on nothing or nobody (Morris, 1991). Although everyone at some point is dependent on someone else, disabled people are marked out as different due to their degree of dependence on others (Oliver, 1990). Thus, disabled people are likely to be dependent on others when it is not expected (Morris, 1991). For example, Morris argues that everyone is dependent on the water companies to provide their household with water but people are only seen as dependent if they need assistance to turn the tap on in order to receive the water. The person needing assistance can only receive it if the other person agrees to carry out the task and does it without drawing unwanted attention to the other person. According to Gignac and Cott, (1998: 740) 'dependency involves both difficulties with a task and a social relationship'. Assistance is dependent on how the interaction proceeds, which involves choice and control. Interdependence focuses on choice and control when requiring assistance (Morris, 1991). Only appropriate choice and control can aid in providing independence. Reeve, (2003) suggests that an inaccessible built environment can cause disabled people to be forced to interact with non-disabled people, including when needing to ask for assistance. This indicates that their dependency could lead to an unwanted situation.

Numerous research has examined the social interactions between disabled and non-disabled people (Goffman, 1963; Hansen and Philo, 2007; Keith, 1996; Scully, 2010). These interactions are often influenced by ableist beliefs, which are evident in how the non-disabled person responds to the disabled person. In his book Stigma, Goffman, (1963) focuses on the issues of 'mixed contacts' which are defined as encounters between the stigmatised (disabled people) and the non-stigmatised (non-disabled people). How a person reacts towards someone with dwarfism asking for assistance is dependent on how that person perceives them.

Although explored in more detail in chapter 4, people's perceptions of dwarfism are shaped by cultural representations, which can impact how people interact with them. Keith, (1996) explores how interactions between disabled and non-disabled people are affected by assumptions and stereotypes towards disability, arguing that interactions are not straight-forward. Social interactions between disabled and non-disabled people can often include subtle forms of disablism. The term 'disablism' was coined to describe all forms of 'discriminatory, oppressive or abusive behaviour arising from the [unjustified] belief that disabled people are inferior to others' (Scully, 2010: 26). Disablism is a product of an ableist society which promotes a particular kind of body and whilst dismissing those who do not match ableist expectations, through discrimination. Keith, (1996) suggests that there are specific cultural rules within society, and although she does not go into detail about what they are, but does include not asking invasive questions or staring, she explains how they are often broken by non-disabled people when socially interacting with disabled people. This, Keith argues, affects disabled people asking for assistance or creates an un-wanted situation when it is provided, as the cultural rules of engagement that enable an interaction to go smoothly are broken.

When exploring social interaction between people with dwarfism and other members of the public, it is important to understand the possible psycho-emotional dimensions of disability (Thomas, 2007; Reeve, 2003, 2006). 'Psycho-emotional disablism involves the intended or unintended 'hurtful' words and social actions of non-disabled people in interpersonal engagements with people with impairments' (Thomas, 2007: 72). Thus, how social inter-actions are played out between people with dwarfism and other members of the public can impact their psycho-emotional well-being.

To reduce unwanted interactions, whilst still being able to interact with space in a way that they want to, people with dwarfism are likely to employ their management strategies, which is an example of a spatial practice. Managing social interactions is a form of agency that permits the disabled person to deal with or overcome a disabling situation. Disabled people are more likely to be more aware of what is going on within the interaction and thus employ a particular management strategy in order to achieve a desired outcome. Relating to Goffman's work on stigma management, Scully, (2010) suggests that dis-abled people often employ their own management strategies, these include:

'normalisation', 'parading' or 'performing'. Normalisation involves down-playing their difference whereas parading involves making the impairment more obvious in order to achieve particular goals, such as receiving assistance or putting the non-disabled person at ease. Performance is used to fulfil non-disabled stereotypes of what constitutes as a particular impairments, which does not necessarily reflect the realities of living with that impairment. Using her own experiences of needing to receive assistance, due to a hearing impairment, Scully points out that it is presumed by non-disabled people that deaf people have a complete loss of hearing, and thus she has to perform as if she is completely deaf in order to receive the assistance she needs. These strategies help to manipulate the non-disabled person's perception of their impairment.

Employing their own management strategies, may allow people with dwarfism to access and interact with a space, however, Scully, (2010) suggests that there is an ethical difference in the encounters between disabled and non-disabled people due to an imbalance of power. It is the hidden labour involved in managing social interactions with non-disabled people, which requires more effort from the disabled person. Scully, (2010) uses the term 'hidden labour' to describe the ways disabled people manage or manipulate the presentation of their impairment to others, due to subtle forms of disablism present within social interactions. The labour is hidden because the non-disabled person is unaware of the work the disabled person is doing, such as manipulation to control the interaction.

3.3 Socio-spatial barriers and dependency

This section attempts to show dependency is socially constructed and that understandings of dependency affect social interactions. Whilst the previous chapter showed the different socio-spatial barriers people with dwarfism encounter, this section demonstrates how these barriers lead to dependency, resulting in different social interactions. To overcome a socio-spatial barrier people with dwarfism may ask for assistance from another person. According to Kittay, (2011: 50) 'assistance is viewed not as a sign of dependence but as a sort of prosthesis that permits one to be independent'. Asking for assistance to overcome a socio-spatial barrier allows a person with dwarfism to carry out everyday tasks, such as shopping. This section explores how experiences of asking for assistance can result in either an enabling or disabling experience, depending on how the other person responds to their request for assistance. Although it is acknowledged that dependency is created by socio-spatial barriers, this section shows that independence is not about having to do a task by oneself but also through receiving the appropriate assistance.

People with dwarfism experience numerous disabling barriers when supermarket shopping, including using a self-service checkout. The self-service checkouts create a situation where a person with dwarfism requires extra dependence on others. Some members of the public may struggle to use the checkouts as they may not be aware of how it works, but for people with dwarfism, it is about being unable to use them due to the checkout's ergonomic construction, which can leave them dependent on others:

> *There is always somebody working there so I actually do that [use the self-service checkout] but the touch screen is too high so I have to ask somebody to assistance me out or ask the person behind me to touch the screen for me (Myraar).*

As the name suggests, self-service checkouts are provided to allow customers to serve themselves in supermarkets. Andrews, (2019: 1) argues that 'in their never-ending quest to further cut costs and boost profit margins, businesses in today's service economy are increasingly turning to self-service'. There is usually only one member or staff in charge of several self-service checkouts, and they are used to assist people for specific reasons, including when purchasing items with a security tag or age restriction, such as alcohol. Thus, the customers still rely on a member of staff to a certain degree but not, for example, when scanning items such as everyday groceries or when using the touch screen to decide what methods of payment to use. A self-service checkout gives customers more independence than they previously had, as prior to their installation people always had to rely on the cashier to serve them, including to scan items and tote up their shopping bill. Not relying on staff as much as they used to means that other members of the public have a higher degree of independence, whereas people with dwarfism are still more dependent on assistance where it is not expected.

Providing people with dwarfism can find someone to assist them still permits them use of the facility, just not in the way expected. Morris, (1999) suggests that independence can come about when a person receives the right assistance. Ensuring that they have assistance still gives people with dwarfism the independence to do their shopping. Receiving assistance can be dependent on a number of factors, including time:

> *... also places where people are very busy and they are not going to consider your needs. Like on a Saturday, I wouldn't even contemplate going shopping then. The shop assistants are busier, and so they can't assistance you as much (Jade).*

The inaccessibility of a place can result in access being restricted to certain times. Jade is restricted in when she can go shopping due to being dependent on others. In this case, it is due to dependency on shop assistants. Jade can feel more comfortable asking shop assistants for assistance as that is part of their job, and they are expected to respond in a pleasant manner. Despite this, Naomi spoke about being refused service at a shoe store and blamed this upon the women being uncomfortable about her dwarfism. Due to companies aiming to reduce staff numbers for cost-cutting purposes, the number of staff available to assistance Jade is likely to be further restricted. Being dependent on others can result in a lack of choice, such as when to go shopping or what items you choose Myraar suggests:

> *Reaching things is very difficult, as I would always have to ask somebody and it is always so difficult because you want to see which item is best, and so you have to wait until another person comes. That can be really frustrating as you don't want to ask a person to keep getting loads of items down for you so you can pick what you want [laughs] (Myraar).*

When a space is created for the average-sized person, it is made to provide the widest range of benefits to them, including the ability to easily reach a selection of items off a shelf. When it comes to certain items such as fruit and vegetables, it is important that people can choose which one they think is best, such as those without bruises. Whereas other shoppers can rummage through items until they find the one they want, shopping for Myraar involves the extra labour of having to keep asking someone for assistance until she receives the items she thinks are best. Otherwise, Myraar just has to take whatever is passed down to her.

In some cases, in order not to have to ask strangers for assistance and thus to be given more choice, people with dwarfism will choose to be accompanied by somebody they know, such as a friend or relative. Taking someone they know means that they can receive assistance when needed:

> *No chance, absolutely no chance. I have tried to use one [self-service checkout] once, luckily enough I was with my sister because I couldn't do a thing … I couldn't reach the screen or chip and pin (Amy).*

> *It would be easier if the counters were lower because then I could go up [to get coffee]. We have never discussed it [her boyfriend], he just automatically goes up, but it would be nice to be able to go up (Alison).*

Creating spaces and facilities, and the facilities within them, without taking particular body sizes into consideration leaves people with dwarfism more dependent on people with the average body size to interact with the facility for them. 80% of people with dwarfism are born to average-sized parents (Little People of America, 2008), meaning that the majority of people with dwarfism will have averaged-sized family members who can assist them with daily tasks. Driedger, et al. (2004) argues that needing assistance, such as from a member of your family, to assist you with a task, such as shopping, is an infringement on a person's independence. It can be argued that being accompanied by someone who is a friend or a relative, who has a better understanding of their needs, will provide better assistance. Being accompanied by a friend or relative allows less reliance on other members of the public, who may be either too busy to provide assistance or who may react in a negative way when assistance is asked for. Scully, (2010) suggests that relying on familiar networks, such as family or friends, reduces the risk of encountering unwanted attention. Although the choice of when to go shopping will be affected by when the friend or relative is available:

> *The desk is too high [post office counter]; it would be difficult to look over ... I'd probably wait another day, go with my parents as they could help me out. I wouldn't ask a stranger as if it's a bank or something, it's confidential and I don't want people knowing my personal details. It's very rare that they have low desks (Jason).*

Jason, who was 24 years old at the time of the interview, has to rely on the assistance of his parents due to the fact that in some cases he is dealing with personal information. Shakespeare, et al. (2010) point out that young people with dwarfism are often more reliant on their parents than those of average stature. If there was a low desk available it would mean he would be less reliant on his parents as he could carry out tasks which are otherwise hindered by a socio-spatial barrier. Despite this, not all people with dwarfism may be able to be dependent on their parents for reasons such as living away from home.

When relying on other members of the public for assistance, it is also about managing the interaction in order for there to be a straightforward interaction. Disabled people often have a range of sophisticated techniques for dealing with other members of the public (Keith, 1996). Monica suggests that this is because people with dwarfism are more socially adept at handling social interactions:

> *I think most people with restricted growth are socially apt because they are used to making first moves with people and having to put them at ease (Monica).*

When a person with dwarfism is shopping alone, they are more dependent on strangers who may be unaware of their need for assistance and may also have their own preconceptions regarding dwarfism. In order to control social interactions when asking for assistance, people with dwarfism will use their own strategies, such as asking for assistance using a particular manner. As Monica points out, people with dwarfism often have to be more proactive with other members of the public in order to put others at ease, people who may otherwise respond negatively to their dwarfism. Disabled people are often more aware of what is going on in social interactions between them and other members of the public (Scully, 2010). Being more attentive to what is going on within social interactions is because people with dwarfism are more aware of how other members of the public are likely to interact with them due to past experiences, and thus making the first move can help to steer a social interaction and avoid any uneasiness.

Managing social interactions is often used to control negative reactions or consequences by others (Taub, et al., 2004). Attempting to minimise any unwanted responses can involve people with dwarfism employing different strategies in order to manage how the interaction takes place, as Naomi points out:

> *I would not be able to reach the carrier bags (Naomi)*
> *How would you overcome those problems? (Erin)*
> *Smile nicely at the shop assistant. Again, it is being able to articulate your needs with a member of staff (Naomi)*

Within her interview, Naomi made it clear that she had a good understanding of how people can sometimes interact with people with dwarfism and some of the ways in which it is best to deal with any unwanted reactions. Goffman, (1963) points out that it is more likely that the stigmatised person has experienced those contacts before and anticipates what the next contact will bestow, resulting in the development of special techniques for dealing with the possible negative social interaction they encounter. This form of stigma management can involve asking for assistance in a particular way, such as smiling nicely. Manipulating a social interaction allows a disabled person to overcome a socio-spatial barrier, in the form of assistance (Keith, 1996). The extra assistance permits Naomi to carry on with other tasks, such as packing her shopping.

Another strategy people with dwarfism use in order to receive assistance with minimal trouble is by making a joke about the situation, as Ivy and Lydia explain:

> *I remember once asking somebody to reach something down, and I made a joke, I'd say, 'everything I want is on the top shelf' ... I don't make a joke of myself to make myself look funny. I do it to make people feel at ease as they are obviously apprehensive about asking me if they can help and so I feel it puts them at ease (Ivy).*

> *I would ask if someone was around. I would make light of it. I would ask them if I could borrow their arm to reach something (Lydia).*

Having to deal with the perceptions of others can be done in a multitude of ways, including the use of humour. Taub, et al. (2004) suggest that using humour can act as a form of deflection, diverting attention away from what they cannot do, diffusing a potentially uncomfortable situation. Making a slight joke about the situation can show the other person that Ivy and Lydia recognise that they are unable to do something due to their height and remove any awkwardness using humour. Schanke and Thorsen, (2014) state that humour in social situations is used by people with dwarfism as a form of stigma management. Furthermore, Shakespeare, (1999) argues that using humour is a way of compensating for any perceived tension or anxiety. Using humour can be used to manage a social interaction by influencing how somebody responds to them when they are asking for assistance. Making a joke in order to receive assistance from another member of the public demonstrates that they are anticipating any difficulties which may be encountered (Keith, 1996). In some cases when a person with dwarfism may need assistance, the cultural rules of engagement can be broken before they have a chance to engage with someone, as Amanda points out:

> *… if I ask people, they will help me if I need something off a high shelf. Although, there was one time when I was standing in Sainsburys [British supermarket], looking at the shelves and this man just stood there next to me and said, 'I bet they get you stacking all the high shelves.' I just walked off, he was trying to be funny and it didn't work (Amanda).*

Even in situations where no communication has been made, some people will still make a comment towards Amanda which may prevent her from asking for any assistance. 'Social encounters are usually governed by culturally agreed rules of engagement' (Keith, 1996: 72). However, the man above ignored these cultural rules of engagement by making a joke about her height. Loja, et al. (2013) comment that non-disabled people often feel that they have the right to intrude and comment upon disabled people. Adding to this, some members of the public also feel the right to joke about a person's bodily difference. Although discussed in more detail in chapter 5, people with dwarfism experience unwanted attention, which is influenced by cultural representations of dwarfism. These representations tend to construct people with dwarfism as humourous and thus create a problematic stereotype of dwarfism. Amanda may have needed assistance but was discouraged from asking as she recognised that the man found her height amusing and asking for assistance from him may have provoked even more unwanted attention. Encounters, such as the one mentioned above, demonstrate that asking for assistance is not a straightforward task, and this can create problems in knowing who to ask for assistance from, as Myraar and Jade point out:

> *I can't do the bagging [at the checkout] so they [cashiers] actually help me out. Sometimes they are really nice, but sometimes they will actually request me to do it myself, but it is so difficult because when they are scanning the stuff afterwards it goes out of my reach (Myraar).*

> *You can only reach the first three levels of a shelf, and so again you have got to engage with somebody to ask for their assistance. A lot of people are assistanceful; some people will ask you if you need assistance. It's such a mixed bag you don't know what to expect on the day. You could one day have some really nice person and the next have somebody say something*

really stupid to you (Jade).

Shopping is becoming more of an independent task due to marketisation. People are expected to be more independent in order for companies to save money. The expectation that a person should pack their own shopping is problematic when checkouts are not accessible. If Myraar perhaps had a more identifiable impairment then assistance would be more straightforward. However, as some people will just view her as small, there is an expectation that she is capable. When deciding *who* is best to ask, in order to minimise the risk of any unwanted attention, this demonstrates that asking for assistance is not a straightforward task. Asking for assistance can only become a straightforward interaction providing Jade or Myraar ask the right person. As Jade points out, there are assistanceful people in society, who will offer her assistance, but then there are others who may say something inappropriate, as demonstrated with Amanda. Ariel also talks about how dependency can be affected by the attitudes of others:

> *I have to keep asking people and, if they are not nice or they don't want to do it, they ignore you or just walk away (Ariel).*

Ariel is widowed and lives in the north of England whereas the rest of her family live in the south of England, leaving her more dependent on strangers. For Ariel there is the extra labour of having to keep asking different people for assistance as she is often ignored increasing the amount of time it takes for her to do her shopping and this can make her feel out of place. Not receiving the assistance needed disables Ariel as she is unable to overcome a socio-spatial barrier. Knowing that asking the wrong person will result in either unwanted attention or no assistance can influence people with dwarfism to only ask particular groups of people within society who they perceive will react in more positive way, such as older people, which Jason points out:

> *The good experiences are when people help me if I need to reach something off a top shelf, in a supermarket, for example. The older generation tend to be a lot more assistanceful as well, so I ask them (Jason).*

Although people's motivations for being assistanceful can be questioned, such as them being able to feel good about themselves (Keith, 1996), within his interview Jason mentioned that older people were generally more helpful and less likely to mock his dwarfism than teenagers. Kittay, (2011) points out that dependency on others involves being able to trust the provider of assistance. This trust is dependent on the type of person that a person with dwarfism judges to be less threatening. Making judgements about people may be related to past experiences, as Jason discussed in his interview about receiving a lot of unwanted attention from teenagers, which is a common experience from other people with dwarfism. Asking only certain people for assistance is a strategy to reduce the risk of unwanted attention. Other people with dwarfism also stated that they would only ask particular members of the public for assistance. As Monica points out, although she is careful who she asks in order to minimise unwanted interaction, she may also purposely ask the wrong type of person in order to change how people respond to her dwarfism:

> *If there is a group of teenagers and I had to choose from asking compared to a relatively young couple or old couple, I think I would choose the couple rather than the teenagers because you know they are going to go off and possibly laugh about it later. On the other hand, I will ask them because actually they see me come out with a normal voice and I am not different (Monica).*

In this instance, Monica, a consultant psychologist, is careful about whom she asks for assistance, due to the risk of provoking unwanted attention. There is a hidden labour involved which requires her to judge how other members of the public may react negatively to her dwarfism. Teenagers often use humour in order to feel part of a crowd, by mocking someone else they deflect any insecurities that they may have about themselves. On the other hand, Monica may consider asking the teenagers in order to take the role of the educator and reduce any unwanted social attention by demonstrating to teenagers that she is no different from anybody else. This is a form of stigma management that challenges preconceived ideas that other people may have about people with dwarfism. In social encounters between disabled people and other members of the public, disabled people often have to take the role of the educator (Keith, 1996). Showing that she is no different demonstrates that Monica is trying to rid any myths or stereotypes that teenagers may associate with her impairment. Davis, (1961) argues that, when disabled people socially interact with another member of the public, their perception becomes 'normalised' and prevents them from treating the disabled person in a negative way. Monica came across as a confident woman in her interview and also when I was recruiting participants at social events; she came across as a bit of an extrovert, which may be why she is more likely to have the confidence to approach people who may react negatively to her short stature.

In conclusion to this section, it is apparent that socio-spatial barriers increase people with dwarfism's degree of dependence on other members of the public. Other members of the public may not have to think about being more dependent on others, providing them with more choice on when to carry out daily activities, such as when to go shopping or to pick up which items they like best. It is not necessarily that their independence is limited, but how assistance is provided that can be disabling. Dependency on other members of the public is not always a straightforward interaction for people with dwarfism, as it involves a more complex social engagement. It is through providing the appropriate assistance and choice that it is ensured that people with dwarfism are still independent within the public spaces.

It is apparent that when asking for assistance the cultural rules of engagement, such as not saying something inappropriate, are often ignored by other members of the public, and this affects the social interactions between people with dwarfism and that public. In order for an enabling experience to take place, people with dwarfism have to employ a range of their own management strategies, showing that they are more adept at controlling certain social interactions. An enabling experience can only come about if people with dwarfism ask the right person for assistance or if they employ their own ways of engagement to make the interaction go without any unwanted attention. What asking the right person further demonstrates is that who a person with dwarfism can ask for assistance is restricted, which means they may spend more time looking for the right person to ask, increasing how long it takes for them to do certain tasks.

When people ask for assistance, it should be recognised that nobody in society is completely independent. Stigmatising dependency, rather than dealing with the fact of and variety of human dependency needs, means we deny disabled people the respect and opportunity to flourish that everyone is due (Kittay, et al., 2005). Considering that everyone in society is dependent at different times, dependence may be more accepted by both people with dwarfism and other members of the public, giving them all better access to spaces and facilities and reducing the need for employing different strategies to receive assistance without any unwanted attention.

Due to people with dwarfism being more dependent on other members of the public and the hidden labour involved in these social interactions, they may opt for finding their own way of overcoming a socio-spatial barrier. This activity lessens their degree of dependency on others. However, doing something differently can result in unwanted attention, such as staring. This can result in psycho-emotional disablism which impacts their decision to overcome a socio-spatial barrier. Changing attitudes would mean that people with dwarfism would not have to employ any extra labour such as, finding the right person to ask or using humour, resulting in a more straightforward interaction.

3.4 Managing socio-spatial barriers

Scully, (2010) suggests that the majority culture, including those of average stature, set normative parameters which all minority groups are measured against, and, in the case of disabled people, includes norms of speech, mobility, pace and so on. What can be added to aid accessability is a way of doing something differently when a disabled person encounters a socio-spatial barrier. People are expected not to take too long carrying out a task and should use a space in the way expected. This is difficult when the materiality of a space is not suitable for your body size. A mismatch in size means that people with dwarfism may take longer using a facility or will employ their own way of interacting with it, for example, climbing on a supermarket shelf. This form of interaction disrupts the normal expectation of behaviour within that space and thus can lead to unwanted social interactions.

This section explores how people with dwarfism manage with socio-spatial barriers and the resultant social encounters. Using their own management strategies demonstrates how they can gain access to the built environment using their own way of doing something. Hansen and Philo, (2007) suggest that spaces have been created for the non-disabled body, and in order for disabled people to fit into these spaces, they have to employ their own way of doing something. People with dwarfism overcoming a socio-spatial barrier in their own way, through using their own managing strategies, can be seen as a form of resistance to a disabling environment. Using a facility differently disrupts the normative parameters in regards to how that facility should be used. Disabled people are often pressured to pass as normal, including using spaces in the way expected (Hansen and Philo, 2007). Using their own management strategies means that people with dwarfism will not be using spaces and facilities in the way expected and this may result in them receiving unwanted attention, suggesting public spaces may be a contributing factor in creating the social restraints, as Monica points out:

> *I think the fact that the difficulty is that sometimes we get looked at more because we are doing things strangely. If you have got somebody of average height where the counter was ten foot tall, then they would be dropping things and doing things that people would look at as it is a bit strange. The environment doesn't assistance us to look normal (Monica).*

Being confronted with a socio-spatial barrier demonstrates that it is not the person's impairment which necessarily makes them act differently, but inaccessible public spaces, and this draws further attention to them. In the last chapter, it was noted that there were many socio-spatial barriers found within a supermarket, such as trolleys being too tall to use. Disabled people often find shopping in supermarkets difficult because of socio-spatial barriers, including difficulties in reaching shelves (Oliver, 1989). Some of these barriers caused people with dwarfism to find their own way of doing something which often attracted unwanted attention:

> *I mean here in Sainsbury's [British supermarket] now where the front of the trolley is quite low, and so I push the trolley from the other way round. It is quite difficult as sometimes they are quite stiff and obviously it is hard. I think they should provide a medium-sized trolley [laughs]. Trolley wise, it is very difficult ... I mean you get stared at but I haven't had any comments (Sofia).*

Turning the trolley around demonstrates a good way of overcoming a barrier, making pushing the trolley easier and giving Sofia more independence to do her shopping. Several people with dwarfism mentioned that pushing a trolley in the way expected was more difficult as it was too big. Pushing the trolley differently results in people staring at Sofia. Chouinard, (1999a) points out that reacting to a person when doing something differently, such as through unwanted attention, marks that person out as negatively different. People with dwarfism are stigmatised, not necessarily because of their body size, but rather because of the lack of accommodations for their impairment. Reacting to a person negatively when they do something differently demonstrates that facilities which are not size appropriate for people with dwarfism cause them to be marked out differently, both spatially and socially. Sofia suggests the solution could be to provide a medium-sized trolley, but supermarkets may not be willing to provide another sized trolley, such as for economic reasons, which is perhaps why Sofia laughs at the suggestion. Despite this some supermarkets are beginning to provide baskets on wheels which may provide Sofia with a more suitable alternative if her local supermarket introduces them. Again, this is dependent on the supermarket's willingness to provide a more diverse range of trolleys, which is unlikely unless it can be deemed that this would increase profits.

In other cases where facilities are out of reach, people with dwarfism have again taken to finding their own way to use a facility, as Lydia and Monica talk about:

> *I can't reach the touch screen and so I end up bashing it with a piece of shopping (Lydia).*

> *If you can't reach to put in your pin number you have to get your purse out and tap it in with your purse or with a ruler that you might have in your bag or a pen. Again, these are all things that make other people look at you because you are doing it different from what somebody would normally do (Monica).*

As discussed previously, self-service checkouts are difficult to use. As a way of using the machine, Lydia and Monica use an item to strike one of the facilities they are using, which can be seen as an extension of their arms making them long enough to use the facility. Having to come up with her own management strategy is a way of overcoming a socio-spatial barrier and acts as a form of resistance to an otherwise disabling facility. The downside is that the situation draws unwanted attention, as Monica mentions, because it disrupts the normal way people are expected to behave within public spaces. This unwanted attention can affect how people with dwarfism interact within public spaces, often restricting them from overcoming a socio-spatial barrier and thus contributing to their disablement. Myraar points out that because of a socio-spatial barrier she has to act differently which causes some people to also react differently to her:

When you are speaking [at a high counter], they can't hear you because the voice thing [microphone] is quite high, and I don't think people realise that and they wonder why you are shouting ... doing something differently leads to more attention and making you look more different and leads to different conclusions as well because I had to speak slowly once so that they could hear me and then somebody came to me and started talking slowly to me and saying, 'Are you alright?' (Myraar).

According to Myraar other members of the public are not aware of how socio-spatial barriers cause her to use her own management strategies, leading them to create their own presumptions about her. Butler and Bowlby, (1997) suggest that the way people with impairments act differently can lead to the assumption that they also have 'impaired minds'. The assumption can result in not receiving appropriate assistance. What can also add to the unwanted attention people with dwarfism receive is how long a task takes to complete, which is often due to the facility not being fully accessible:

You can't reach in [dip tray in a bank] because they are so deep. If it is something you are doing frequently they get used to you and they recognise how it is acceptable for you to do it ... They are wondering why you are taking longer and that naturally draws attention (Amy).

In this case, as Amy points out that taking longer to do something draws attention to the situation as the normal speed is disrupted, but becomes acceptable over time as people become used to her situation. In society there are not only expected ways of doing something but expected time limits. However, if you are having to struggle to reach something this will undoubtedly add more time it takes you to carry out a task. For example, imagine being in a queue at a checkout and the person in front is taking a long time to pay for their goods. Unless you understand why they are taking longer to pay you would eventually become impatient. Past experiences indicate that you only take a few minutes to pay for your items, unless there is an acceptable reason not to. It is up to others to recognise this and accept that for people who are having to interact within a space that is not ergonomically suitable for them, then they will take more time. Similarly, Myraar encounters the same problem when using a chip and pin machine:

If you request them [chip and pin machines], they can take them out for you but there have been moments where they can't take them out and have to call other workers to help take it out. It causes a big scene so people who are shopping there are staring and wondering what is happening and they all know it is because I can't reach something (Myraar)

Being unable to access the chip and pin machine brings unwanted attention to Myraar's inability to reach the facility as opposed to the inability of the member of staff to remove the chip and machine. Taking longer to do something acts as a hindrance to the normal speed of doing things and is seen as wasting time (Hansen and Philo, 2007). Kayleigh faces a similar situation which limits how often she will visit a particular supermarket:

> *... they are bolting the card machines to the card holder, and I need it passed down to me ... I have noticed at Morrisons [a British super-market] here, I have stopped going a lot and will only go occasionally, and it is because I can't be arsed faffing about with their card readers ... Yeah and it makes me feel very self conscious as people have lined up innocently behind me and, then the queue begins to get massive, and although I know it is not my fault but rather Morrisons for bolting their things unnecessarily to counter tops, you do become self conscious (Kayleigh).*

The way in which particular facilities are constructed and where they are placed often results in them being inaccessible, even more so when a facility is not adjustable in height. Wendell, (1996) points out that disabled people often take longer doing something than is normally expected and this can cause unwanted attention. For people with dwarfism, their unusual body size already provokes unwanted attention, and thus the added, unwanted attention created by inaccessible infrastructure can exacerbate the psycho emotional disablism they already experience. Attracting more attention because of how long it takes to do something makes Kayleigh, in this si-tuation, self conscious and has prevented her from going to this particular supermarket as often as she used to. The reactions from other members of the public, coupled with the struggle she has using the facility, limits Kayleigh's access to a particular space. Not using their own management strategy may also be dependent on space and time, as Amanda and Naomi point out:

> *I can get on to bar stools but I am conscious that I am making a spectacle of myself as I get on and off (Naomi).*

> *... in some places, such as pubs, all the chairs are really high and they are a nightmare to get on. I can get on them but it attracts a lot of attention from drunks who find it funny. If it was busy, then I would not bother trying to get on the bar stool, but if it was quiet I would (Amanda).*

Amanda is aware that she is going to attract a lot of unwanted attention if she uses her own way to get on a high chair. The ergonomics of a particular facility creates a situation which involves Amanda both struggling with a socio-spatial barrier and a social restraint. Attracting unwanted attention can be affected by time and space. During particular times, certain spaces are likely to be busier, such as a pub during the evening. As pointed out in the majority of interviews, a lot of people with dwarfism receive unwanted attention, including comments and jokes towards their height, particularly from people who have been drinking. Shakespeare, (1999) argues that social rules of engagement are often broken when people are inebriated. To overcome this Lydia suggests making light of the situation:

> *Do you find getting on the bar stools can bring negative attention? (Erin)*
> *No, I make light of it. I find if you feel there is going to be some negativity maybe due to an embarrassment because of the way you do something in a different way. If you make light of it or raise the attention of it before you do it, then the embarrassment is taken away (Lydia)*

The social restraints in these cases are outweighed by the person's wish to sit on a bar stool which, because of a mismatch in size, they have to get on differently. Morris, (1991) argues that in order for disabled people to gain acceptance within society, they need to emulate normality. Doing something differently does not emulate normality and can therefore draw unwanted attention. However, making light of the situation should lessen any discomfort which may arise because of doing something differently (Taub, et al., 2004). This is a form of resistance to any unwanted attention which may be encountered. Lydia has to manage the situation, through deflecting any embarrassment, and she does this through making the situation seem less important than what it is and reducing the chance of anyone else passing comment. Lingsom, (2011) points out that responding to a disabling situation in a positive way is used in order to be accepted within the company of others. Joan and Steve talk about how they are more reluctant to do something in their own way if a place is crowded:

Erin:	*Do you find that if you have to do something differently you might not do it if there is a crowd?*
Joan:	*Yes.*
Steve:	*Just avoid it.*
Joan:	*Leave it there.*
Erin:	*Do you think that if it didn't grab attention you would do it?*
Steve:	*Yeah. In some instances when we are on a coach or something we take a footstool.*
Joan:	*A little plastic stool.*
Steve:	*People even watch you doing that. Even that sort of attracts attention … Anything that is not the norm is something they look at. I wouldn't say they can't accept it but it is something different for them.*

Joan and Steve indicated in their interview that since being together they have noticed that more people stare at them. For example, if they were shopping and Joan was further down the aisle than Steve, he would notice people staring at Joan. Anything they have to do differently Joan and Steve point out attracts unwanted attention, in the form of staring. In a crowd there is going to be a higher potential of attracting attention from an individual or several individuals than there is in a smaller group. It is not only socio-spatial barriers which restrict access to different spaces but knowing that accessing particular spaces, such as crowded spaces, will be dominated by stares and other forms of unwanted attention (Morris, 1991). The staring occurs because, as Steve suggests, anything that is different from the norm attracts the attention of others. Not doing something differently is a strategy to limit how much unwanted attention they both receive, especially as they are already very aware of how much unwanted attention they both receive because of their already visible impairment. Refraining from using their own management strategy may limit unwanted social attention, but it causes them not to be able to overcome a socio-spatial barrier, causing disablement. As Lydia points out, if attitudes towards people doing something differently were more positive, more socio-spatial barriers could be overcome:

> *People's attitudes and the way they treat you can override the environment. Say, for instance, you couldn't access something because of your height, if the people that are around you had a positive attitude and they could see a way around it and alternative route for you then, you are there. It doesn't matter if that physical environment was not accessible as long as there are positive attitudes around you could overcome it (Lydia).*

Although changing the physical structure of public spaces helps to improve access for disabled people, including people with dwarfism, changing the attitudes and behaviours that other members of the public have towards disabled people can also provide better access (Butler and Bowlby, 1997). Better social attitudes will aid in reducing psycho-emotional disablism and make them feel like more accepted members of society.

This section has explored the different management strategies people with dwarfism use to overcome socio-spatial barriers. As public spaces are created for a narrow range of people, only they can access them in the way expected. Within this section, it is apparent that people with dwarfism employ a number of their own management strategies in order to be able to carry out different tasks, such as being able to use a self-service checkout independently. The way of overcoming a socio-spatial barrier reduces how physically disabling public spaces are for people with dwarfism and permits them to be more independent. Scully, (2010) suggests that managing social interactions is a form of agency.

People who do not conform to what is average in terms of appearance or behaviour are no longer 'normal' (Morris, 1991). As dwarfism is a very visible impairment, it can be suggested that doing something differently further differentiates people with dwarfism from the norm. Doing something differently is likely to provoke an unwanted reaction from other members of the public and can be treated with suspicion or hostility (Hansen and Philo, 2007). This section has shown that what can prevent people with dwarfism from overcoming a socio-spatial barrier are social restraints, which are dependent on time and space. Different spaces attract different people and provoke different behaviours, such as a pub which is going to be busier on a Saturday night and full of people who are under the influence of alcohol, as opposed to on a Monday morning.

The expected way of doing something is not just dependent upon how the task is done but how long that task takes to be completed. Not completing a task in the time expected can be blamed upon how that facility is constructed, which can make them inaccessible for people with dwarfism. In both situations, the management strategies that people with dwarfism use lead to unwanted social attention. Accepting what Hansen and Philo (2007: 493) call 'the normality of doing things differently' would allow people with dwarfism to overcome a socio-spatial barrier, giving them increased access to different spaces and the facilities within them. It is about making people aware that spaces and facilities can be used differently and that there should be no set way of doing something. It is not just their body size that provokes stares but also doing something differently.

Whilst people with dwarfism often receive unwanted attention for doing something differently, they also showed that they were experienced in dealing with the situation. Having to employ their own management strategy relates to Goffman, (1963) and Scully, (2010) who suggest that interactions between disabled and non-disabled people require the disabled person to employ their own management strategy in order to deal with a possible negative social interaction. This is a form of hidden labour that could be eliminated if the causes of disablism were challenged.

3.5 Conclusion

This chapter has explored the different ways in which people with dwarfism respond to socio-spatial barriers, including through dependency on others or using their own management strategies. Social restraints can affect people with dwarfism asking for assistance or deciding to overcome a socio-spatial barrier in their own way. The findings in this chapter add to Keith's (1996) argument concerning disabled people's encounters with strangers, including through floating cultural rules of engagement. Dependency on others and doing something differently ensure that people with dwarfism can access different spaces. Avoidance may be due to not wanting to draw attention to themselves if they have to interact with a barrier in their own way in order to overcome it, or avoidance might be because they are concerned about the response from others if they ask for assistance.

Whilst a person with dwarfism's degree of dependency is affected by physical barriers, the social interactions are affected by social norms and values surrounding dependency and how tasks should be done. A person with dwarfism's degree of dependency aids in demonstrating how disabling public spaces are for them. Altering different spaces and facilities would reduce their dependency and permit them to use facilities in the way expected. As an accessible built environment is not always possible, Scully, (2010) points out that if disabled people have to ask for assistance then the social encounters involved would have to be free of any embarrassment or hostility. As shown people with dwarfism are often accompanied by a friend or family member when shopping, suggesting that familiarity provides an easier interaction.

4 Disabling identities

4.1 Introduction

As demonstrated in the previous chapters, people with dwarfism have to negotiate spaces that are created for the average-sized person, which results in numerous disabling situations. Although considered to be a disability (Kruse, 2010), including within the American's with Disabilities Act (1990), dwarfism is often contested as a disability. This raises the question, what do people consider to be a disability and how does this affect people with dwarfism? Dwarfism is often seen more as a difference than a disability. This is due to a number of factors, including the lack of recognition of body size as a disability.

The identity of people with dwarfism as disabled people is important to consider, as it can provide access to accessible spaces, as well as other disability services, including welfare. It is important for people with dwarfism to be able to access these amenities as they aid in providing better equality. Obviously, not all disabled people consider themselves disabled and this choice is important to respect. However, it is also important to explore the reasons they may not consider themselves disabled and why that may be problematic.

The first part of this chapter provides a review of the various literature in relation to disability perceptions, including arguments surrounding body size and disability. The first analysis section of this chapter focuses on the social interactions between people with dwarfism and other members of the public when requiring access to accessible spaces. As recognised in chapter 2, accessible spaces can be more accommodating than their non-accessible counterparts. This is because some of the facilities within these spaces are placed lower in comparison to their non-accessible counterparts and thus are more appropriate for people with dwarfism. This shows how a change in the statuarization of a space makes it accessible for people with dwarfism. However, the materiality of a space is not enough to make it fully accessible. This section demonstrates how the representation of a space is also an important aspect of access. The representation of accessible space is constructed by disability stereotypes, which can impact upon who can access the space. Wendell, (1989) suggests that how society recognises disability can affect those who they do not perceive as disabled both socially and economically. Depending on whether people with dwarfism are perceived to be a disabled person can affect their access to accessible spaces, as they first must match the representation of the space. This section explores some of the interactions between people with dwarfism and other members of the public when trying to access accessible spaces.

Building from the previous analysis section, the second analysis section explores how attitudes towards people with dwarfism change when they use a mobility aid, such as a wheelchair or mobility scooter. This section gives a better understanding as to how different disabled people are perceived and some of the resulting implications for people with dwarfism. It exposes a hierarchy of impairments, which favours those with more recognisable impairments. This is not to imply that people who use a mobility aid do not encounter disablism within society, but it gives a more nuanced approach to how different impairment groups are treated.

With contention within society regarding dwarfism's identity as a disability, it is important to explore how this impacts upon a person with dwarfism's self-identity as a disabled person. Drawing on the notion of 'internalised ableism' the last section explores whether people with dwarfism identify themselves as a disabled person and the reasons why, including how their perceptions of disability reflect different understandings of disability.

4.2 Disability identities and body size

A criticism of the social model relates to its origin. The social model was developed by disabled activists who all shared the same or similar impairments (Shakespeare, 2004, 2013). Most of the activists had physical impairments, but dwarfism was not one of them. Who the social model was developed by, Shakespeare, (2004) suggests, affects other impairment group's inclusion within the disability community and leads to a narrow understanding of disability. Whilst Shakespeare recognises the benefits of the social model, he also argues that a narrow understanding of disability does not fully combat disabled people's social exclusion due to their complex needs. As shown in chapter 2, accessible spaces only provide access for a narrow range of disabled people. It can be argued that the origin of the social model has aided in providing a more inclusive built environment through the implementation of accessible spaces, but on the other hand it has also created a false representation of accessible spaces, which is influenced by a narrow perception disability.

Issues relating to a disability identity, including the importance of recognition as a disabled person have been explored mostly in relation to those with invisible impairments (Rhodes, et al., 2008; Stone, 2005; Sutherland, 1981; Wendell, 1989, 1996). Stone, (2005) and Rhodes, et al. (2008) explore how having an invisible impairment creates problems in terms of being recognised as a disabled person, especially in relation to reactions from other members of the public as there are no markers of disablement. Problems include not being seen as a disabled person and as a result being expected to carry out tasks which they are unable to do or being denied access to accessible spaces. However, dwarfism is a very visible impairment, but this does not mean that they are recognised as disabled people. It is the recognition as opposed to the visibility of an impairment that can prevent access. In this case, the lack of recognition of body size as a disability.

Geographies of body size questions if fatness is a disability, (Brandon and Pritchard, 2011; Chan and Gillick, 2009; Cooper, 1997; Herndon, 2002; Kirkland, 2008; Longhurst, 1997, 2010). Longhurst, (2010) suggests that there are similarities between fatness and disability in relation to spatiality as the materiality of spaces are often disabling for fat people due to the size of spaces being created for people with a lower body weight. Cooper, (1997), Chan and Gillick, (2009), and Kirkland, (2008) point out that a lack of understanding of the social model of disability by other members of the public affects their perception of what disability can be. Similar to dwarfism, fat people have to negotiate spaces that are not size-suitable for them.

Numerous research within Geographies of body size explores how the sized body interacts with, and experiences spaces (Colls, 2004, 2006; Evans, et al., 2012; Hopkins, 2012; Longhurst, 2005, 2010). Spaces that are not created for a particular body size can be related to the social model of disability, whereby minority forms of embodiment are excluded from the built environment. Longhurst, (1997, 2005) points out how elements of the built environment such as narrow stairs and small changing rooms, form spatial barriers for people with large bodies. However, this lack of access tends to be ignored. Cooper, (1997) and Longhurst, (2010) also suggest that fatness is not considered a disability as it is seen as blameworthy whereas disabled people are deemed non-blameworthy for their impairments. This argument cannot be applied to dwarfism as in most cases the cause is genetic. Thus, the reason why dwarfism is contested as a disability is more complex.

4.3 Social encounters within accessible spaces

It is fair to say that people with dwarfism are often lacking from disability imagery. The majority of images that depict disability access, such as within information leaflets, booklets and stock images used in the media for newspaper articles on disability are dominated by wheelchair users. There seems to be no room for other impairments, including dwarfism. Sutherland, (1981), focusing on disability stereotypes and definitions, argues that disability is mainly understood as being unable to walk, and this is signified by the presence of a mobility aid. This creates a very homogenised and misleading representation of disabled people. Due to the wheelchair and wheelchair users being the dominant representation of disability, other disabled people often experience difficulties in being recognised as disabled (Morris, 1991; Moshe and Powell, 2007; Reeve, 2006; Sutherland, 1981). Dominant representations of disability are used to signify the presence of an accessible space or facility. Most accessible spaces, including accessible toilets and parking spaces, are represented by the International Symbol of Access (ISA) (Figure 4.1).

According to Lydia, the ISA is not fully representative of disabled people:

The stick person in a wheelchair [ISA] only represents between 5 and 8% of the total population of disabled people, so the logo is wrong (Lydia).

Lydia works for a disability organisation, which is probably why she showed a sophisticated understanding of disability issues. Although impairments requiring the use of a wheelchair are more common than dwarfism, less than 10% of disabled people living in the UK use a wheelchair (Sapey, et al., 2005). The ISA is probably the most widely recognised representation of disability. It is a pictorial symbol which allows it to be used internationally, as it can bypass all linguistic barriers. The ISA denotes that access has been provided for disabled people and that only disabled people may legitimately access that space (Moshe and Powell, 2007). Society understands that accessible spaces should only be used by disabled people and thus to access an accessible space, a person must first have an identifying signifier of disability, such as mobility aid.

The ISA produces a homogeneous representation of the disabled population, which Morris, (1991) and Sutherland, (1981) argue creates a false stereotype of disability. As a result, both Ivy and Monica think it is the reason other members of the public fail to consider people with dwarfism as disabled people:

Why do you think people wouldn't consider you to be disabled? (Erin)

Well because the disabled symbol is a wheelchair and they always think it

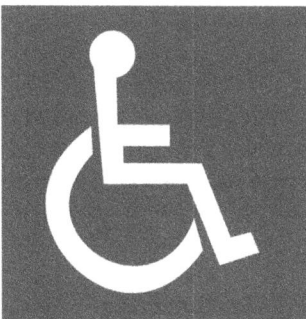

Figure 4.1 International symbol of access. (Stock Image)

is people in a wheelchair. (Ivy)

> *The sign for disability is somebody in a wheelchair. I don't think people know whether to categorise us [people with dwarfism] as disabled (Monica).*

The ISA supposedly represents access for all disabled people yet it is an image of a wheelchair user which only represents a specific group of disabled people. The symbol implies that disabled people are visibly recognisable by their use of a wheelchair. Furthermore, in their report, Shakespeare, et al. (2010) argue that the disabling effects of dwarfism, including medical and social aspects, are not always apparent. Secondary impairments, such as spinal stenosis, remain invisible, not just in the literal sense, but as shown in the next chapter, they remain absent within cultural representations of dwarfism. Consider how many charitable adverts you have seen, asking for donations to help disabled people and how many of those feature someone with dwarfism. This is not to imply that people with dwarfism should be included within charity adverts, as these come with their set of problematic stereotypes, however, they do help to promote who is disabled. The failure to include people with dwarfism within media images of disability further adds to their lack of recognition as disabled people.

A very recognisable accessible space, which is marked by the ISA, is the accessible toilet. The ISA influences the representation of this space and its representational space to others. Accessible toilets are often found in various spaces within the built environment, but they are often segregated from the non-accessible toilets. The segregation of the accessible toilet from the other toilets makes it more recognisable and indicates that is for a specific user. Despite various impairments being able to benefit from using the accessible toilet people's perceptions can determine who can use them without question. As Chouinard, (1999a) suggests, not fitting the disabled stereotype can result in unwanted attention, including being questioned when trying to access accessible spaces. What makes access difficult are assumptions from other members of the public. As Jade points out, the ISA resulted in her being challenged by a wheelchair user when requiring valid access to the accessible toilet:

> *I had a wheelchair user tell me off once for using an accessible toilet because I wasn't in a wheelchair. I explained how I couldn't reach the sink, the lock, the dryer or see the mirror. She still didn't think that they were also for us, because that symbol seems to say that it is specifically for them (Jade).*

When interviewing Jade, she demonstrated a clear understanding of how the built environment is disabling, and she spoke about a number of her own disabling experiences due to her dwarfism. Jade's need to use the accessible toilet is due to the number of facilities in which the non-accessible toilet is too high for her to use. Despite this, she points out that the wheelchair user did not recognise her needs, only her own, which was supported by the ISA. The ISA symbolises the woman's impairment, not Jade's, and thus she failed to realise that the accessible toilet provides access for a range of disabled people. The ISA is often placed prominently on the entrance door of the toilet, indicating that it is only for disabled people and only they may enter that space. The problem is the meaning of the space is distorted by problematic imagery. The ISA creates a common problem for disabled people who are not wheelchair users as they are often policed when using an accessible space or facility (Moshe and Powell, 2007). People's perception of who can legitimately use the accessible toilet overrides the aim of the space, which is to provide access for any disabled person. Reeve, (2006) suggests that people who do not match the stereo-typical image of a disabled person, which is often a wheelchair user, can result in their right to access an accessible space being disallowed. Naomi mentions being disallowed from an accessible space which could have otherwise alleviated a disabling situation:

> *The other problem is when you go to rock gigs is that you go into the disabled platform if you are in a wheelchair, but I am the same height as somebody in a wheelchair, but they won't let me because I am not in a wheelchair (Naomi).*

Naomi spoke in her interview about how she was a fan of Bon Jovi, a popular rock band, and sometimes went to their concerts. Article 30 of the United Nations Convention on the rights of persons with disability recognises the importance of being able to participate equally with others within cultural activities, including access to cultural venues (United Nations, Article 30, 2006). However, equal access is dependent on the recognition of who is disabled. The UN may have encouraged the representation of cultural spaces to change, i.e. including an accessible space, however, the representational space conceived by the staff impacts Naomi's access. Both people with dwarfism and wheelchair users require access to the accessible area in order to be able to see over the crowd, but clearly the member of staff only saw the wheelchair users as needing alternative access. Not allowing Naomi access flouts Article 30 of the UN's convention on the rights of people with disabilities. It also ignores Naomi's self-identity as a disabled person, which produces an ableist power relation whereby the non-disabled person gets to decide who is and is not disabled.

Furthermore, not only does being in a crowd make seeing the band difficult but it can also pose a safety risk. Kruse, (2010) states that people with dwarfism tend to avoid large crowds as they can be easily shoved or knocked to the ground due to their height and lower body weight. If Naomi had been granted access to the disabled platform there would have been less chance of her being knocked or shoved, thus increasing her safety, as well as allowing her to clearly see the band. Being disallowed from accessing a space due to not using wheelchair calls into question what other members of the public perceive disability to be. Other people's perception can result in people with dwarfism actively avoiding an accessible space:

> *You said you went to a concert in Wembley [stadium] and didn't use the disabled area. Why did you not use it? (Erin)*
> *Because I didn't really, I didn't prefer to go to it, but it was just the first time I had ever gone, and me and my partner just went. I suppose I just prefer to be treated as normal, but you could see it and it was just mainly full of people in wheelchairs and maybe they [people in charge] wouldn't ... wouldn't ... they probably wouldn't have understood because I am not in a wheelchair or something. You're not disabled, you know. (Tracy).*

The representation of a space influences Tracey's spatial practice. Tracey avoids using the accessible space at a concert, partly because she wants to be treated in the 'normal way', denying her the use of a space which may give her better access. This is a form of internalised ableism, which favours normalcy and thus stigmatises the non-normative way of being. People with dwarfism are often reluctant to identify with the wider disability community (Shakespeare, et al., 2010). Sitting with the other disabled people, would re-inforce Tracey's identity as a disabled person. The next section shows people with dwarfism do not always consider themselves disabled. Tracy also avoids attempting to access the space because she assumes that the people in charge would not be aware of her needs, presuming that they only see wheelchair users as disabled, which is dependent on the staffs' interpretation of that space. People who are disabled by the built environment, but who are not recognised as a disabled person, are often expected to perform in the same way as non-disabled people (Wendell, 1996). Challenging staff can be tire-some, as it involves a form of hidden labour, which is not always met with success. Being disallowed or challenged is because, according to Monica, people are unsure whether dwarfism is a disability:

> *If you go to a normal counter they never think about going to the low counter and serving you there. Again, I think it is about people not quite knowing whether we are disabled or not (Monica).*

A low counter is a more suitable alternative to the regular counters, as it is low enough for someone with dwarfism to see over it, allowing for better communication between them and the member of staff. It will also allow the person with dwarfism to be able to use the desk to sign any papers and to transfer any documents to the member of staff. It is not enough that accessible spaces are implemented, but that people recognise that they can benefit a number of users who would otherwise struggle. The inability for staff to provide reasonable accommodations for people with dwarfism can be attributed to a lack of disability training, which does not include the needs of people with dwarfism. However, common sense should indicate that a person with dwarfism would be better off using a low counter. Many people assume that accessible spaces are solely for wheelchair users, despite the fact that they benefit other disabled people (Moshe and Powell, 2007). A low counter is used by somebody in a wheelchair, not because the person has a mobility impairment, but because being in a wheelchair reduces their stature, as they are in a sitting position as opposed to a standing one. Thus, the purpose of the low counter is to serve someone who is shorter and this should obviously include people with dwarfism.

Spaces being unsuitable due to a person's bodily difference would, of course, correspond to the social model of disability that places the cause of disablement within society and the built environment. Instead, it can be argued that body size is not considered a disability because it is not a functional limitation on the body which is often apparent with the addition of a cultural marker of impairment, such as a wheelchair. In most cases, people with dwarfism feel that if they were a wheelchair user they would not have any difficulty in accessing accessible spaces. In spaces where there is only one low counter, but several other regular counters available, it can mean that a person's probability of ending up at the one low counter is unlikely, which Amanda further discusses:

> *What about if there was only one low counter? (Erin)*
> *I wouldn't be guaranteed it in the queue and I am not in a wheelchair so I couldn't just go up to it. (Amanda).*

Other people's perceptions of a disabled person, which Amanda thinks is a wheelchair user, denies Amanda guaranteed access to the low counter. 'One stereotype is that you're either in a wheelchair and helpless or on your own two feet and capable' (Sutherland, 1981: 1). People with dwarfism and wheelchair users share a common experience which is that both of them require access to lower facilities due to an otherwise un-accommodating built environment. Whilst Amanda's need to use it is the same as a wheelchair user, she presumes she does have the same right of access. This presumption influences the representation of a space and thus does not make it fully accessible for all disabled people. It may not be that people understand a wheelchair user's needs, but that accessible spaces are for the sole benefit of wheelchair users, and people with dwarfism who use these spaces legitimately are seen by other members of the public as fraudsters trying to reap the benefits that these spaces offer, such as no queuing. Kayleigh, on the other hand, chooses to directly to the low counter:

> *I had it at the train station because there was only one low counter for wheelchair 'users', so I lined up and that meant I jumped the queue because there was a queue of fifty people for twenty desks but there was only one desk which was low, so I had to line up behind the low desk. The woman said, 'I am sorry madam but there is a queue'. I told her that I was only able to use her desk because if I line up with everybody else I actually end up lining up twice as long because all the other desks are inaccessible so I have to let people go past and use them and wait for the low counter to become free. It is the same in the post office as well. (Kayleigh).*
>
> *Somebody was saying that before that you are not guaranteed that when it is your turn you are going to get the low counter. Do you think it would be different if you were in a wheelchair? (Erin)*
>
> *Yes. They would automatically see it as the wheelchair counter as opposed to the disabled counter. (Kayleigh).*

Kayleigh, who showed a lot of confidence in her interview, openly challenged the member of staff who did not recognise her need to use the lower counter despite Kayleigh being only 3′ 2″ tall (96 cm). Instead the member of staff accused Kayleigh of queue jumping because, as Kayleigh suggests, people recognise the counter as a counter for wheelchair users and not for someone with dwarfism. This demonstrates that it is acceptable for Kayleigh to wait in line and allow people to go before her, but it is unacceptable for her to go before them and use the one counter which is size-suitable. The member of staff's response may at first just seem ignorant, but it is a subtle form of disablism which results in inequality which is exacerbated by other difficulties people with dwarfism experience when in a queue. Being in a queue can be an undesirable experience for people with dwarfism as they are often given a lack of personal space by other members of the public, and in some cases are unable to stand up for long periods of time due to mobility impairments. Being able to go straight to the low counter would therefore help to alleviate the problems of queuing, as well as allowing them to use a counter ergonomically suitable for their height. Whilst Kayleigh challenged the situation, some people are more reluctant:

> *… A year or so back, I went into my bank and I went to the low counter, and the woman called across and she said, 'we have got no staff there, you'll have to come up to one of the others'. I dealt with the person I had to deal with and he said, 'sorry about that'. I didn't say anything, but when I got home I wrote a letter and said that I had got embarrassed because I went to the low counter, and I know I am not in a wheelchair but it is ideal for me, and I was told to go to another one. I got a phone call and an apologetic letter saying that I should have said I want to be served here and they would have got somebody. Once again that would have all caused attention (Ivy).*

The staff's unwillingness to accommodate for Ivy's impairment demonstrates the unequal power relation between Ivy and the member of staff. The member of staff who is situated at the non-disabled, higher counter, would have had to move to the lower counter, which seems to be an inconvenience for her. However, for Ivy, having to interact with a counter that is too high for her is not so much an inconvenience but is a disabling experience. The member of staff having control over that space constructs Ivy as inferior. As Ivy's situation demonstrates the staff's reluctance to adhere to providing disability equality results in the extra labour of Ivy having to fight for access by explaining her needs. Taub, et al. (2004) suggest that in order for disabled people to receive disability assistance they must first assert the existence of their disability. Ivy could not just walk in and choose to use a facility more suitable for her, but first had to prove her need for it because of the staff's ableist attitude. This involves some extra labour for an activity that should usually be straightforward. Having to confront an average-sized member of staff can be intimidating for someone of short stature and can lead to an unwanted interaction. Writing a letter removes Ivy from the situation, which may have caused a scene, but still allows her to fight for appropriate access and shift the ableist power relation.

4.4 Becoming 'Truly' disabled: using a mobility aid

Disabled people are not one homogenous group that experiences the same forms of disablism within society. There may be similarities, such as being stared at or being asked intrusive questions. However, different impairment groups receive different unwanted attention. Every impairment comes with its own set of attitudes and stereotypes within society (Tringo, 1970). These stereotypes and attitudes can affect how different disabled people are treated in society. This is not to try and compete as to which impairment group is treated worse in society, but to understand why some may encounter more social barriers than others. By noticing the differences, the reasons can be easier to locate and combat.

Particularly in middle-age, people with dwarfism experience pain and stiffening in their joints and back, and, in the case of those with Achondroplasia, they may experience spinal stenosis, restricting their mobility (Shakespeare, et al., 2010). Due to these secondary impairments, some people with dwarfism use a wheelchair or mobility scooter in order to access public spaces. What is interesting is that when people with dwarfism use a mobility aid, how other members of the public respond to their presence changes. Joan and Steve point out that when they use a mobility scooter they believe they receive less unwanted attention:

> ... *We have got electric scooters and use them in pedestrian areas. If we are walking we get stared at, but if we are on the scooters nobody looks (Joan).*
> *So you find you get less attention when using a scooter? (Erin)*
> *Yes (Joan).*

> *Why do you think that is? (Erin)*
> *I've heard others who use a wheelchair also say it. They don't get as many stares (Joan).*
> *You're just another disabled person (Steve).*

It cannot be ignored that just because they use a mobility scooter they are not stared at, but as Steve points out, he and Joan are stared at less. Tringo's (1970) hierarchy of impairments demonstrates how society favours some impairments more than others. A lot has changed in terms of disability equality since Tringo first established the list of impairments in order of favour within society, however, this insight demonstrates how there is still a hierarchy of impairments, as attitudes towards people with dwarfism change when they use a mobility aid. Even in more recent studies on hierarchies of disability, dwarfism still remains low in terms of acceptance, whereas impairments that require the use of a wheelchair, such as paraplegics, remain more acceptable. Smelkin argues that the more visible an impairment is, the less desirable it is within society. Of course, a wheelchair user is a very visible person with an impairment, however, it is not usually their bodily appearance that is different. Typically, a wheelchair user is an average-sized person in a wheelchair, whereas a person with dwarfism is someone with profound short stature and a disproportionate body size. There are of course many wheelchair users who do not have a normative body, however, it is the wheelchair that is usually the first thing people see, which is a signifier of disability as opposed to someone who carries the cultural baggage of dwarfism.

When using a wheelchair, Joan and Steve's body size and shape are less visible, and the wheelchair becomes their main identifier. Garland-Thomson, (2009: 161) suggests that 'perhaps the most spectacular form of visual novelty that can prompt stares is breaches of common human scale and shape'. Furthermore, people with dwarfism are an uncommon sight and carry an identity which links them to the mythic and low brow entertainment, which constructs them as spectacles (explored in more depth in the next chapter). This is not to suggest that the visibility of their dwarfism completely disappears but that the first thing other members of the public are likely to see is their mobility aid, which changes the identity of someone with dwarfism. Wheelchair users are more socially invisible than people with dwarfism as they are a more familiar sight within society and tend to be ignored (Shakespeare, et al., 2010). Between 1986 and 1995 there was a 100% increase in wheelchair users in England and Wales, which is partly due to an aging population (Sapey, et al., 2005). However, it is also the number and types of comments which change when a person with dwarfism uses a wheelchair. Alison points out that she receives fewer comments when using a wheelchair:

> *... Patronising comments whereas if I am in the wheelchair I get that less. I think people don't notice that I am a little person as much (Alison).*

Keith, (1996) argues that wheelchair users often do receive patronising comments from other members of the public and that people with a physical impairment are often infantilised. The fact that Alison receives fewer patronising comments when using her wheelchair may be related to her small stature that is not as visible when she is sitting down and her wheelchair being more visible. It is not uncommon for people with dwarfism to receive patronising comments due to their small stature. Shakespeare, et al. (2010) and Kruse, (2002, 2010) point out that because people with dwarfism are the same height as a child they tend to be infantilised, especially women with dwarfism. Patronising comments were especially apparent for people with dwarfism who do not have Achondroplasia, such as Alison, and therefore do not have a different body shape. Not having a different body shape means that they are just small in appearance and perhaps more closely resemble a child in appearance. Not surprisingly, the less unwanted attention they receive when using a mobility aid results in them feeling like a more accepted member of society:

> *When I am on the scooter, I am treated differently; I am a more accepted member of society, than when I am not using it (Jade).*

Jade spoke about how she received a lot of unwanted attention which could make her feel out of place. Wheelchair users may be more socially accepted especially since impairments with a bodily difference, including dwarfism, are often devalued (Dear, et al., 1997). It is not suggested that wheelchair users do not receive any unwanted attention within public spaces. Lenney and Sercombe, (2002) point out that wheelchair uses are often prone to stares from other members of the public, but that there is a hierarchy of impairments, which is influenced by cultural representations of different impairment groups and the rarity of some impairments within society. Although explored in more depth in chapter 5, it must be considered that cultural representations of dwarfism are an influencing factor in how they are treated within society. Despite this, Jade did talk about an incident when she was using her mobility scooter which prevented her from getting on a bus to access the town centre, as the bus driver would not allow her to go on with her scooter. Although when in public spaces she may be treated in a better way, it is not to be ignore that there are still negative attitudes aimed towards someone using a mobility scooter which can also restrict access to spaces, such as on public transport.

4.5 Disabled or not disabled?

As shown in chapter 2, public spaces can be disabling for people with dwarfism. Despite this, not all people with dwarfism consider themselves to be a disabled person. This section shows that the self-identity of a person with dwarfism is influenced by different understandings of disability and can result in internalised ableism. Taub, et al. (2004), Shakespeare, (2006), Watson, (2002) and Wendell, (1996) note that disability is often associated with stigma and stereotypes, including helplessness. Negative connotations to disability can affect the self-identity of a person as disabled (Vernon, 1996). Nobody wants to admit to having an identity which is stigmatised within society.

An important factor to consider when focusing on self-identity as a disabled person is whether a person has a social or medical model understanding of disability. People with dwarfism often see themselves as being like any other member of society except shorter (Ablon, 1990). The irony about only seeing themselves as shorter and not disabled is that their shortness in public spaces created for an average-sized person is disabling. However, a medical model understanding of disability would ignore the disabling impact of the built environment and would instead conceive disability as a functional limitation, often associated with pain. Ariel does not consider body size to be a disability:

> I am disabled because of my legs … but if I was just like you [meaning being of small stature] no (Ariel).

It is only with the addition of problems with her legs, which is a result of her dwarfism, that Ariel considers herself to be disabled. It is Ariel's pain in her legs, which impedes her mobility, which she sees as disabling. Ariel does not include body size as a disability despite her mentioning in her interview a number of disabling barriers she encountered within the built environment due to her small stature. Although it was in the 1970s that disability began to be understood as being caused by disabling barriers caused by society and the built environment, it was not until the early 1990s that this understanding became more prominent (Barnes and Mercer, 2010). At the time of the interview, Ariel was 54 years old, and her ideas of disability reflect a medical model understanding of disability which has had and continues to have a strong influence on how disability is conceived.

As shown previously, dwarfism is not always recognised as a disability within society and this can affect whether or not people with dwarfism identify themselves as a disabled person. Reeve, (2006) and Stone, (2005) point out that self-identity, as a disabled person, is affected by interactions with other people:

> Do you consider yourself to be disabled? (Erin)
> That is a very hard one. At work we have an access network which is for disabled people. Up until last year, I never ever ticked a box to say that I am disabled. I am in a way, yes, but there is never anything that covers me, I am not blind, deaf or unable to walk (Charlotte)

A lack of recognition of body size as an impairment on a form at work affected her in identifying herself as disabled which could affect her receiving the appropriate support needs. The impairments mentioned are all functional limitations on the body, resonating more closely with a medical model understanding of disability. Charlotte spoke about how when growing up her parents never talked about her dwarfism and that she was expected to act as if she did not have dwarfism, including by not having any adaptations made to her family's home. Schanke and Thorsen, (2014: 1467) point out that 'families not openly talking about having restricted growth as differences or otherness, was part of a normalisation strategy. Silence may have been the most available option to avoid transmitting concerns about abnormality and cultural taboos to the child'. 80% of people with dwarfism are born to average-sized parents (Understanding Dwarfism, 2013). It is likely that these parents have specific perceptions of dwarfism based on cultural representations of both disability and dwarfism. Added to this, according to France, et al. (2012), most expectant parents choose to end a pregnancy when they discover the foetus has an impairment. This is not to suggest that children with dwarfism are not wanted but that it is hard for some parents to accept their child's dwarfism. These attitudes are influential to Charlotte's internalised ableism. Internalised ableism is defined by Campbell, (2009: 7) as a means to emulate the norm, the disabled individual is required to embrace, indeed assume, an 'identity' other than one's own. If Charlotte had recognised herself as a disabled person, she may have been entitled to disability support through her network at work, which would have placed her on a more equal standing with her colleagues. Claiming a disability identity can prove beneficial as Lydia points out:

> *Would you consider yourself to be disabled? (Erin)*
> *I use and abuse it. I use my disability to my advantage. If it is to my advantage, then yes I am disabled. If it is not to my advantage, then no I am an able-bodied person (Lydia)*
> *Would you consider yourself to be disabled? (Erin)*
> *To get me first in the queue at Disneyland because I can go on the fast track queue. Somebody will offer to do something for me instead of me having to do it. Certain benefits that you can get, price reductions because you are disabled, you use and abuse it (Lydia)*
> *When would you not consider yourself disabled? (Erin)*
> *When I am having a good day and I am not reminded that I am a dwarf and I feel at one and I am enjoying life (Lydia)*

There are, according to Lydia, costs and benefits to claiming a disabled identity, which shows that Lydia's identity as a disabled person is fluid and dependent on different circumstances. Rhodes, et al. (2008) suggest that identity is fluid and is dependent on the various understandings of disability. Accepting themselves as a disabled person means that people with dwarfism further differentiate themselves from other members of the public. Ablon, (1990) suggests people with dwarfism are often reluctant to consider themselves as a disabled person because it means adopting another label, as they are both someone with dwarfism and a disabled person. Choosing when to adopt a disability identity means they are more in control of their identity and can make disability seem like a positive identity if it comes with benefits. Although Lydia classes dwarfism as a disability, she also associates dwarfism with negativity which she relates to socio-spatial and social barriers that she spoke about in her interview. Lydia also only mentioned that she was reminded of her dwarfism when she received unwanted attention. The negativity associated with dwarfism and disability can be the cause of internalised ableism. These barriers of course would relate to the social model of disability which shifts the blame from the person to public spaces and considers social interactions to be disabling. Shifting the blame to society and the physical structure of public spaces means that the fault is not with her body. Lydia's refusal of a disability identity, unless positive, is a form of stigma-handling that aids in providing her with a normal identity the rest of the time. Schanke and Thorsen, (2014) claim that people with dwarfism find it important to preserve a normal identity that demonstrates that they are just like everybody else. Similarly, Amy is reluctant to class herself as disabled:

> *What do you think disability is? (Erin)*
> *Not being average. Not being part of the norm (Amy)*
> *Would you consider yourself to be disabled? (Erin)*
> *Different (Amy)*
> *Why? (Erin)*
> *I am a little person. I am a Mum. If anybody asks me what I do I say that I am a Mum. I am the same as any other Mum, and I do all the Mum things like washing and ironing. I class [names her son] as disabled because he can't do things for himself. I think if you can do things for yourself and you can carry out day to day life then you are just different. If you can't do anything without the aid of somebody else you are disabled (Amy)*

A disabled person is someone who deviates from the norm in terms of social expectations, whether this is in terms of mobility, sight, or in the case of dwarfism, height. Dasen (1988) points out that dwarfism is over three standard deviations below the mean height of the population. This would then make dwarfism a disability in relation to Amy's suggestion that disability is not part of the norm. However, Amy classes herself as different as opposed to disabled despite her claim and pointing out a number of socio-spatial barriers she encountered within public spaces. This again resonates with internalised ableism, where Amy rejects a disability identity as it is associated with negative values, such as dependency. Amy points out the other identities she has, including being a mother, overrides a disabled identity and indicates that she is capable and that others are dependent on her. Other social roles, such as being a mother, makes disability insignificant (Watson, 2004). Amy also considers her son who has severe cerebral palsy to actually be disabled as he is unable to carry out everyday tasks which Amy can. Schanke and Thorsen, (2014) point out that people with dwarfism consider themselves 'normal' as they have the ability to carry out everyday tasks, which makes it difficult for them to accept a disability identity. However, as shown in chapter 3, people with dwarfism are often dependent on help from others when carrying out everyday tasks, such as shopping. Her degree of dependency differs in the sense that she is less dependent than someone with a more severe impairment, such as cerebral palsy, but more than a non-disabled person. Kennedy, (2003) explains that it is common for people with dwarfism not to see themselves as a disabled person and that they will usually compare themselves to other people with impairments, such as wheelchair users, in order to deny their disability. Comparing themselves with other disabled people allows them to play down the disabling effects of dwarfism:

> *I wouldn't see myself as disabled although I can't do as much as most people, but I have a friend who has Muscular Dystrophy, and I can do more than her as I can do more for myself. I think little people are more independent and somebody disabled can't do as much as us. A lot need constant care like someone to do their shopping or drive them about (Sofia).*

> *What do you think disability is? (Erin)*
> *It's something that someone has wrong with them, either in a physical, mental or emotional capacity. I suppose you would say it was a permanent problem that somebody has (Jennifer)*
> *Would you consider yourself disabled? (Erin)*
> *Yes, I suppose I would as I am not able to do absolutely everything. However, this is where society has that problem of putting that label onto people. I am ten zillion times more able than somebody with limited use of their arms or legs or in a wheelchair. You cannot say that I am disabled in the same description as them (Jennifer)*

Comparing themselves to other disabled people neglects that there are various severities of disability, but instead constructs disability as something which is severe and often viewed from a medical model perspective. This may be due to the stigma attached to being disabled, as disability is often represented in a negative way within society. Lenney and Sercombe, (2002) suggest that disability is often viewed negatively as it is associated with debilitating effects. Having an identity which is perceived negatively can, of course, lead people to deny it. Often disabled people compare themselves with someone less fortunate in order to enhance their self-esteem (Deal, 2003). Despite both Jennifer and Sofia encountering socio-spatial barriers within public spaces, they avoid fully recognising themselves as having a disability and use examples of other disabled people to play down their disability status. This Morris, (1989) claims is a form of internalising oppression which includes some people with impairments approximating themselves more closely with what is considered normal in terms of appearance and abilities, whilst differentiating themselves from those who do not.

Whilst some people with dwarfism are reluctant to class themselves as a disabled person, others recognise that dwarfism could be disabling. Myraar suggests the built environment disables everyone at different times and in different ways:

> *What do you think disability is? (Erin)*
> *I think it is a short-term or long-term effect for a person. It either can be a mental thing or a physical thing that stops somebody from doing something that they like to do and leading a life like most people do (Myraar)*
> *Would you consider yourself to be disabled? (Erin)*
> *That is actually a very good question. At certain times I think we are all disabled in some way. I think even average-height people are disabled at certain times in their life. I think if I can't do something then there is always some form of access. If I can't reach something high up like a switch, I can get a chair and switch it on. Certain other things like not being able to reach the alarm on the tube then yes I feel very disabled (Myraar)*

Myraar works as a special needs coordinator and considers disablement something to be when there is no way of overcoming a physical barrier. Within her interview, Myraar spoke of many alternative ways to overcoming socio-spatial barriers which would reflect Hansen and Philo's, (2007) assertion that disabled people have different ways of interacting with a built environment which is not suitable for them. It is only when these barriers are impossible to overcome that Myraar considers herself disabled, in the same way she points out that everyone is, showing reluctance to being seen as different from other members of the public. Similarly, Alison and Kayleigh consider themselves to have a disability due to inaccessible spaces and also because of having to do things differently:

> *What do you think disability is? (Erin)*
> *I am very much of the social model of disability where disability is caused by society. If everything was accessible there wouldn't be disability. Yes, there would be … no, there wouldn't be really any disabled people because we would be enabled and not disabled anymore. I think disability is also caused by people's perceptions as well because people's perceptions and their prejudice, they're the ones that label us. If we were seen as the same*

as everybody else in society, we wouldn't be labelled. I also see it as someone that does things differently that may look a bit different, but at the end of the day we are all the same (Alison)
Would you consider yourself to be disabled? (Erin)
Yes (Alison)

What do you think disability is? (Erin)
I think it is a combination of both the medical and the social model. I think that a body does deviate from a certain standard and more commonly occurring norm which gives disability so, for example, if you can't walk, you are disabled as most people can walk, however, the degree to how much you are disabled by that is socially determined. It is about planning and design and social attitudes which are disabling. I think it is very presumptuous of the medical model to presume that somebody wants to be fixed (Kayleigh)
Do you consider yourself to be disabled? (Erin)
Yes. I consider myself to be disabled leaning more towards the social model because I do believe that my biggest barrier is social attitudes as well as building design (Kayleigh)

Alison's suggestion that society creates disablement for people with dwarfism reflects a social model point of view. Alison and Kayleigh also recognise that society's attitude towards dwarfism contributes to their disablement. Kennedy, (2003) points out that dwarfism is a 'social disability' as people with dwarfism do encounter a lot of unwanted attention which can impact their well-being. These factors are disabling as they prevent access to various spaces, including accessible spaces. Monica, despite being reluctant to class herself as a disabled person, also blames the built environment for creating disability:

What do you think disability is? (Erin)
I don't think anybody is disabled. I think the World is disabled for them. If the World was for us, you know, like if I got out of bed in the morning and the bed was only 6 inches off the floor and only 4 foot in length and the ceilings were only 5 foot and I could see out of the windows then I wouldn't be the one who be disabled, people of average-height would be disabled. To me, I don't see disabled people. I see the World as disabled (Monica)

Would you consider yourself disabled? (Erin)
I would consider that the World is disabled for me (Monica)
Why? (Erin)
Practically and physically things aren't made for us and that we have difficulties negotiating this World (Monica)

Monica's definition of disability reflects a social model understanding. Shifting the blame to society, or the 'World' in Monica's case, shows that the problem is not with Monica's body but rather how public spaces have been created to exclude her. Monica's explanation for considering herself to be disabled by socio-spatial barriers would reflect Finkelstein, (1975) suggestion that creating public spaces to suit a particular group of people disables another and thus it is them which create disablement. Finkelstein argued that by creating a house to solely accommodate for a wheelchair user would disable somebody who was not a wheelchair user. In the same way, creating a place which was ergonomically suitable for people with dwarfism would disable anyone who is over 4' 10" (147 cm) tall. However, there are solutions, such as Universal Design, which consider the needs of a wide range of users. People with dwarfism can be accommodated by providing multi-level and height-adjustable facilities, which would not be disabling for other users. In a similar way, Jade takes into account both a social and medical model understanding of disability:

> *What do you think disability is? (Erin)*
> *It is having a medical condition which limits some of the things you can do. That is a small part of it though. The major barriers are attitudes towards us, lack of housing, transport, bad media representations. This needs to be challenged because they all stop me from doing things and that's what disability is. Disablement means to stop and to stop you from doing something (Jade)*
> *Would you consider yourself disabled? (Erin)*
> *Yes, I am disabled by the built environment and by society's lack of understanding and awareness (Jade)*

Jade takes into account both a medical model and social model understanding of disability, but mostly considers public spaces and attitudes towards her dwarfism to be disabling, including the media, much of which will be explored in the next chapter. This understanding resonates with the social model of disability. Limitations caused by secondary impairments can include mobility difficulties, and, in the case of Jade, this is also brought on by having osteoporosis. This places a restriction on the amount of activities Jade can do, including leisure activities. It is, of course, important to take into account 'impairment effects' (Thomas, 2004). Impairment effects can include pain, which of course can restrict people with impairments pursuing leisure activities.

This section has shown that there are mixed feelings about people with dwarfism considering themselves to be disabled. A number of factors, including their own understanding of disability, influences a person's self-identification as a disabled person. An understanding of the social model of disability results in more people self-identifying as a disabled person, whereas a medical model understanding, which is often associated with negativity results in fewer people with dwarfism considering themselves disabled. People are often reluctant to class themselves as disabled as it is often perceived as a stigmatising social label (Shakespeare, 2006). Comparing themselves to other disabled people with more severe impairments justifies their belief of not being disabled. Not recognising themselves as a disabled person can be related to ableist assumptions of what is considered 'normal'. Campbell, (2008) suggests that in order to emulate the 'norm', which in this case is the able-bodied, average-sized person, the person will recognise others as disabled. This Campbell, (2008) points out is a form of internalised ableism which recognises people's acceptance of the norm as being that of the perfected body which is free from disability.

Perceptions of disability and thus their acceptance as a disabled person is influenced by the different models of disability. Shakespeare, (2006) suggests that within society there is still a lot of ignorance surrounding the social model of disability as many people are unaware of its existence. People with dwarfism who showed an understanding of the social model of disability were more inclined to class themselves as a disabled person. Using the social model of disability people with dwarfism are disabled. Adopting a social model understanding of disability shows that there is something wrong with public spaces as opposed to their bodies. Oliver, (1990) argues that by shifting the notion of disability from the person to society shifts the understanding of normality from the person to society and thus society is viewed as abnormal. A lot of people with dwarfism have a negative view towards disability, which affects their acceptance towards recognising themselves as a disabled person. Blaming public spaces or comparing themselves to someone with a more severe disability plays down a disability identity and makes them appear more normal.

4.6 Conclusion

This chapter has shown that a hierarchy of impairments exists and is created in different ways. People with dwarfism create their own impairment hierarchies in order to dismiss a disabled identity. It reinforces the belief that only particular people with impairments are disabled. This may be reinforced by the experiences many people with dwarfism have encountered within society, such as being challenged when trying to access accessible spaces. The different understandings of disability influence other members of the public's perception of dwarfism as a disability. Dwarfism is often not considered to be a disability by some other members of the public, which impedes upon their access to accessible spaces. This difficulty results in disabling barriers not being fully alleviated. Recognising dwarfism as a disability can help to create a more inclusive society. It is not enough to change the physical structure of spaces; social attitudes must also change. An inclusive society can only come about if everyone, regardless of the impairment, is given access to public spaces and this includes access to accessible spaces.

Attitudes towards different impairments differ, as they change when people with dwarfism use a mobility aid, resulting in a hierarchy of impairments. This is not to suggest that people who use a mobility aid do not receive unwanted attention, but that there are hierarchies which are influenced by various factors, including the rarity of dwarfism and also how it is culturally represented. Cultural representations of dwarfism are explored within the next chapter and, as shown, differ significantly from stereotypical representations of disability.

5 Cultural representations of people with dwarfism and the social consequences

5.1 Introduction

This last analysis chapter explores how cultural representations of dwarfism, including historical and present day representations in popular culture, including mass media, socially construct people of dwarfism. Popular culture is defined as 'All those elements of life which are not narrowly intellectual or creatively elitist and which are genuinely although not necessarily disseminated through the mass media' (Hinds, et al., 2006: 2). Mass media includes television, advertising, films and newspapers. These forms of mass media are broadcasted to a large audience. It is estimated that worldwide 1.67 billion households own a television (Watson, 2019). Furthermore, there were 176 million cinema admissions in the UK in 2019 (Johnson, 2019). When exploring cultural representations of dwarfism, it is important to consider how these representations construct people with dwarfism in wider society and the social implications.

According to Ablon (1990: 885), dwarfism is 'a physical difference [that] also carries with it historical and cultural baggage that has created a mythic stereotype'. This chapter explores how social attitudes towards people with dwarfism are influenced by cultural representations and what strategies people with dwarfism employ to deal with them. It is argued that cultural representations of disability play an important role in shaping the everyday disablism that disabled people encounter. Disablism is prominent within society in many different forms, including through cultural representations, which can shape how disabled people are perceived and treated within society. Disablism can be associated with human dignity. A lack of dignity renders a person inferior within society, which is a key component of disablism.

In order to understand the impact of cultural representations of dwarfism, it is important to engage with the views and experiences of people with dwarfism. The first part of the chapter explores how people with dwarfism think their impairment is culturally represented, including some possible positive representations of dwarfism. This provides a nuanced exploration of representations of dwarfism, which aid in understanding how people with dwarfism perceive different representations. Whilst dwarf entertainers are often given a vast amount of attention, very little is known about the consequences of their actions. This chapter aims to give a voice to people with dwarfism who are not in the limelight but experience the repercussions from those who are. Kennedy, (2003) argues that dwarfism is a social disability. The second part of the chapter focuses on the wider social implications, which influence the spatial practices of people with dwarfism. Different spaces will have different meanings, or representations, which can influence different responses towards people with dwarfism. For example, a cinema showing a film featuring a character with dwarfism is likely to prompt a negative response to someone with dwarfism occupying that space.

The last part focuses on how people with dwarfism think dwarfism can be depicted within the entertainment industry. This aids in giving them a voice, which for centuries has been silenced by average-sized producers and writers, as well as a minority of dwarf entertainers. A more positive representation of dwarfism will aid in challenging problematic stereotypes, which in turn should aid in changing how people socially engage with people with dwarfism. Improving social interactions can aid in providing people with dwarfism better access to the built environment, changing their spatial practices.

5.2 Cultural representations of dwarfism

Cultural representations of disability play an important role in influencing disablism within society. Research concerning disability representations, in relation to the media, includes children's literature and disability (Blaska, 2004), disabling images in advertising (Haller and Ralph, 2006), the portrayal of disability on television (Backstrom, 2012; Sancho, 2003; Wilde, 2007), the cinematic representations of disabled people (Darke, 1998, 2004; Norden, 1994; Wilde, 2018) and disability representations used for charitable purposes (Barnes, 1991b, 1992; Morris, 1991; Shakespeare, 1994). Barnes, (1992) suggests that disabled stereotypes within the media, including on television and in films, create assumptions about disabled people and thus affect attitudes towards them in society.

Dwarfism has strong links to the entertainment industry. Shakespeare, et al. (2010) point out that people with dwarfism are very prominent within popular culture, including mass media, and suggest that there is a cultural fascination with them. Throughout history to the present day, people with dwarfism have been sought after as entertainers and as curiosities due to their bodily appearance (Backstrom, 2012). The *Journal of Literary and Cultural Disability Studies'* special issue on representations of dwarfism (2020) provides an in-depth exploration of how people with dwarfism have been represented in various forms of media and during various historical eras, from biblical times to 1930s cinema. Pritchard and Kruse, (2020) argue that it is important to explore how people with dwarfism are represented within cultural texts in order to understand the way they are conceived and perceived within society. Adelson, (2005b) provides a chronological account of the lives of dwarfs from Ancient Egyptian times to the present day. Dwarfism's history includes court jesters, freaks, pets for European royalty, being depicted as mythological creatures and public spectacles (Adelson, 2005b). In European courts, people with dwarfism were often kept as pets to emphasise the status of the royals. The ability to keep a dwarf as a pet demonstrates their inferiority within society. Although it is claimed that dwarfs kept by royalty had a better life than others did (Woolf, 2019), it results in a lack of power and agency on their behalf. Tuan, (1984, cited in Adelson, 2005b) points out that court dwarfs were constrained by dominance, whilst being indulged and exploited. Their destiny was constructed and controlled through disablist attitudes of those with power. Whilst they were probably indulged, this was through the control of the average-sized keeper, as opposed to being able to create their own destiny. In the 18th century, European courts began to decline, however, people with dwarfism became sought after for freak shows.

The Victorian freak show is one of the most well-known historical shows which exploited those with bodily differences for profit. As Gerber (1993: 435) suggests, the 'exhibition of people with bodily differences, also known as freaks, is a form of social oppression and exploitation which contributes to the reproduction of the prejudices and discrimination that people who bodily abnormalities face'. One of the most famous performers of the freak show was Charles Stratton, better known as 'General Tom Thumb'. This name automatically creates an incongruous encounter, whereby his title suggests that he is a high-ranking military official, whilst his name denotes his small stature. However, (Woolf, 2019: 189) points out how 'Tom Thumb was described by Punch magazine as a joke of nature. He was laughed at as he was deemed unthreatening and unfitting'. Although the freak shows are now practically nonexistent, it is important to note that people with dwarfism are used in other forms of entertainment that are a form of exploitation that has disabling consequences for people with dwarfism in society.

When the freak shows began to diminish, the film industry became another way to exploit people with dwarfism for the amusement of others. People with dwarfism are prominent in films such as Tod Browning's *Freaks* (1932), *Snow White and the Seven Dwarfs* (1937), *The Wizard of Oz* (1939), *Austin Powers: the Spy who Shagged Me* (1999) and Austin Powers in Goldmember (2002), *Time Bandits* (1981), *Willow* (1988), *Willy Wonka and the Chocolate Factory* (1971) and *Charlie and the Chocolate Factory* (2005), where their dwarfism is their main feature and is played upon in a comedic or fantasy way. Gerber (1993: 50) points out that 'whilst there have been few film or television roles available to them, those that have mostly dwell on their dwarfism and fail to present them as ordinary human beings'. Watson, (2020) argues that the depiction of people with dwarfism in 1930s cinema reflected the representation of dwarfism within the freak shows. Furthermore, Bolt, (2019: 32), in reference to Tod Browning's Freaks, argues that the 'freaks were defined by their non-normative embodiment rather than complex characterisation. Many of the disabled characters have minimal or no dialogue, as if the actors were not employed for their talents but exhibited for visual effect'. This can be applied to numerous films where all of the characters played by dwarf actors are given limited dialogue, but their dwarfism is prominent, similar to a freak show exhibition.

In several of the films, people with dwarfism are depicted living in separate societies (see *Wizard of Oz and Willy Wonka and the Chocolate Factory*). According to Wilde, (2018), people with dwarfism are viewed as a separate race, which is reinforced within the media. The depiction of several people with dwarfism living together further enhances the exhibition of their non-normative body. Seeing one person with dwarfism is enough to evoke fascination, however, several together is even more of a spectacle. Yet, in reality most people with dwarfism will find themselves being the only person with dwarfism living in their local area. Rarely is someone with dwarfism depicted as an ordinary human being, or someone with an impairment, but rather a mischievous being, happy to be ridiculed and always to be laughed at rather than with. Whilst these stereotypes abound in books and films, which help to separate them from fiction and the real world, other representations of dwarfism bring these fictional representations to life.

Beside films, dwarfs are also prominent in lowbrow entertainment which provide close interaction between them and their audiences. It is almost as if the fictitious representations people have been exposed to have been brought to life. Adelson, (2005b) points out that since 1999, as a result of online publicity, demand for dwarf entertainers has increased. People with dwarfism are popular in lowbrow entertainment, including as nightclub performers and as someone you can hire out for a celebratory event. For example, there are various agencies that 'hire out' dwarfs for entertainment purposes, such as 'The MiniMen' and 'Cheeky Events' based in the UK. A quick look at Cheeky Events' web page indicates that dwarfs are acceptable figures of fun:

> *Cheeky Events are one of the very few agencies that can provide you male or female dwarfs for rent. What you need them for, or would like them to do, is entirely up to you (within reason of course!), but our clients often use them for promotions, singagrams or as waiters or even for wind-ups (Cheeky Events, 2014).*

In the same way the freak show allowed audiences to gaze at an extraordinary body, firms such as Cheeky Events allow their clients the chance to be entertained by dwarfs or more specifically by their dwarfism as opposed to any talents. All of the activities imply that dwarfs can be used to provoke a humorous reaction from those who have rented them out. Adelson, (2005a) points out that casting adverts for people with dwarfism often advertise height as a prerequisite for the role, but talents are not required. Some dwarf entertainers may call themselves 'professional entertainers' but many are simply spectacles used to encourage disablist behaviours from the average-sized audience who relish in laughing at the performer's deformed body. This can be considered a form of internalised ableism, whereby the dwarf entertainer is adhering to disablist representations that are exploitive and oppressive.

Dwarfs are not only available for hire, but similar to the depiction of dwarfs living in groups, they have often been placed in groups for entertainment purposes. Adelson, (2005a: 4) points out that 'well into the 20th century, sideshows, midget villages and travelling troupes performing musical extravaganzas were popular, perpetuating the illusion that happy communities of very short people were a naturally occurring phenomenon. Midget villages that appeared in western society in the 20th century provided a way for people with dwarfism to be deemed a spectacle. Midget villages have not so much disappeared, but have rather arisen in other parts of the world under different names. In 2009, the 'Kingdom of Little People' opened in China, where the one and only attraction are people with dwarfism, who all live in the Kingdom and dance on stage for the average-sized visitors. All performers are housed in fairy-like structures, which reinforces and brings to life the mythological stereotype associated with dwarfism. The Kingdom segregates them from the rest of society and further encourages them to be perceived as a novelty. The Kingdom is reminiscent of the midget villages that were a byproduct of the freak shows (Howells and Chemers, 2005). The Kingdom has generated some controversy, including being branded a human zoo, however, the average-sized owner, Chen Mingjing claims that the place helps people with dwarfism to escape discrimination and find employment. This is despite China's disability laws that aim to provide access to employment and equal opportunities for disabled people to engage within society. The Kingdom of Little People only further reinforces discrimination experienced by people with dwarfism through constructing them as a novelty.

5.3 How people with dwarfism think they are culturally represented

This part explores how people with dwarfism think their impairment is culturally represented. Dwarfism is often represented in an unrealistic way, as Jade points out:

> ... *They [people with dwarfism] were always in a circus or in a scary film as part of the horror genre. We were something to be laughed at or something to be scared of, there were no short people who were just short. There were no short presenters or newsreaders, there was nothing (Jade).*

An absence of people with dwarfism in ordinary roles indicates that they are misrepresented in the media. Only representing dwarfism as something scary or funny creates a distorted view of the people that differs significantly from an ordinary person, leading an ordinary life. In relation to disability in horror films, Bolt (2019: 27) introduces the term '*horrification*' to describe the 'potential for a non-normative social aesthetic that is identified but represented in a way that induces fear'. This indicates that using a dwarf in a horror film is because their distinctive body size and shape can provoke fear, rendering them scary. Being perceived as either funny or scary is stigmatising. Something scary is to be avoided and thus not part of society. Representing dwarfs as either funny or scary is problematic due to the rarity of dwarfism, as there is limited opportunity for people to encounter people with dwarfism leading ordinary lives. If the majority of representations present a fictitious view of people with dwarfism, then other members of society will have a distorted view of them. Barnes and Mercer, (2010) point out that disabled people when on television are not depicted as ordinary members of society, including an absence of them in roles, such as newsreaders. Although Jade speaks in the past tense referring to when she was a child, Lydia and Ivy go on to mention how present day, humorous representations of people with dwarfism are influenced by past representations:

> *I think the clown in the circus era is where the ridicule and making fun of has come from because you were a clown in a circus and you were made fun of and ridiculed and you were there to be made fun of and laughed at. I think we have an almost difficulty in letting go of that ridicule because of the historical references back to circus times (Lydia).*

> *…, you always saw a small person in the circus and the circus is something you go to laugh at (Ivy).*

In the circus, dwarfs often played, and continue to play, the role of clowns, which are well-known comedic performers. 'Clowning provides a general conceptualisation of dwarfism in the British circus tradition' (Carmeli, 1988: 130). In places such as circuses, people were encouraged to humour and mock performers such as people with dwarfism, but pity was always absent (Bogdan, 1996). A history of people with dwarfism being objects of ridicule indicates a strong link between the impairment and humour and not a passing phase that is likely to be easily forgotten. 'Dwarfism is a very visible impairment, with many connections to comedy and the circus in our culture' (Shakespeare, 1999: 48). According to Lydia, there is an acceptability to laughing at people with dwarfism. Laughing at people with dwarfism is a form of disabling humour, which renders them inferior.

This humorous construction of dwarfism is also prominent within television shows. Amanda refers to a British sitcom, supposedly based upon the life of someone with dwarfism, however, the main character with dwarfism is encouraged to be laughed at and ridiculed:

> *I have recently seen that trailer for that show [Life's Too Short] with Warwick Davis [dwarf actor]. It's meant to show a dwarf's life but he gets stuck in a toilet, how is that a dwarf's life? I have never known that to happen. It's just having the fun made out of his height (Amanda).*

The portrayal of people with dwarfism as humorous differs significantly from their actual life, creating a false impression of them. *Life's Too Short* debut achieved 2.5 million viewers (Halliday, 2011). What Amanda talks about is a situation that is very unreal, unlikely to happen and yet something that provides a supposedly humorous situation. Even in the present day, people with dwarfism continue to be represented in a degrading manner (Kruse, 2010). This degrading representation is a form of disabling humour, which uses the dwarf body to provoke laughter and robs the person with dwarfism of any dignity. Dignity is often associated with humiliation and degrading treatment (Kaufmann, et al., 2011). In relation to dwarfism, this usually comes under the guise of humour. The fact that the show first aired in 2012, indicates that this is a modern day representation that shows that the connection between dwarfism and humour is still prominent. Alison further points out how dwarfism is still shown as humorous:

> *I think the times where in programmes where you have just got a little person there just because they are a little person and for no other reason just to make fun of them. I know there was a children's programme that was on within the last few years, and there was a little person just there to be laughed at. Well, actually I have just remembered another one, there was another children's programme that was more recent, and the little person was there as a baby. He was dressed up as a baby and was in a baby's pen, so they were just there because they were little and they weren't there just because they were like any other person in society. I think that is wrong because that then gives people the impression that it is ok to laugh at little people because they are like that on the TV (Alison).*

Alison makes it clear that, according to her, the characters with dwarfism that she has seen on television are used as a source of amusement because of their appearance, which reflects the use of people with dwarfism within the freak shows. Alison mentions two children's programmes where people with dwarfism were used to be ridiculed, which she believes could encourage children to think that they are a source of entertainment and acceptable to laugh at. Kruse, (2003) points out that a child's early references for people with dwarfism, such as fairy tales, can blur the boundaries between what is real and imaginary for a child. These representations could encourage unwanted attention from children. Alison mentions that a person with dwarfism was used not to represent another member of society, more appropriate for his age, but is instead infantilised due to his height. Bolt (2014) refers to the treatment of disabled people as children as 'disablist infantilisation'. Disability infantilisation is problematic as it constructs people with dwarfism as inferior and permits them to be treated in the same manner as children. Kruse, (2003) states that it is frustrating and insulting for someone with dwarfism to be infantilised. Treating an adult as a child demeans their social status and can affect how seriously they are taken, including when working in a professional occupation.

Amanda further talks about how in films or on the television the focus is still on the height of someone with dwarfism, which is constructed as humorous:

> *We [people with dwarfism] always seem to be something you can mock and make fun of because we are different. We are humorous and different and that's ok … We are still being laughed at. People still see us for our height and nothing else. Most of the time when we are on TV or in a film the focus is on our height and nothing else (Amanda).*

According to Amanda, there is an acceptance towards making fun of people with dwarfism. Even today, people with dwarfism continue to be used in various entertainment venues, usually more for appearance than talent (Adelson, 2005b). The height of someone with dwarfism is the source of entertainment opposed to any talents that he or she may have, such as being a good actor or singer. The fact that they are only used due to their appearance indicates that their height is entertaining, especially as it is encouraged to be laughed at. Similarly, Jason mentions how people with dwarfism are only used as a source of humour:

> *You're [people with dwarfism] always the funny person, never the person taken seriously. It doesn't matter what film it is, the small person is always laughed at …. Say for example in a movie they tend to be mocked in a way, they are more of a joke than a serious part in the film. They don't have a serious side to them, they are always the funny ones (Jason).*

Their body size and in most cases body shape is read as something funny and never to be taken seriously. Darke, (1998) argues that films help to construct stereotypical representation of disabled people that misrepresents their actual lives. Films are watched by a wide audience and thus it is important to take their significance into account when focusing on social attitudes in relation to disability. Adding to this, Naomi talks about how even in a film with limited comedy appeal, characters with dwarfism are still represented as something to be laughed at:

> *… Even if you look at* Lord of the Rings *[popular book and film trilogy], I loved* Lord of the Rings *but there is no mention of dwarf throwing in the*

book but there is in the film when Grimly [dwarf character] asks Legolas the elf, 'I can't jump that gap you'll have to toss me'. I am very familiar with the work of Tolkien [author of Lord of the Rings*] and there is no mention of dwarf tossing in Tolkien's work, but that was used as a comic thing in the film for the audience and lets be honest* Lord of the Rings *isn't full of comedy (Naomi).*

The Lord of the Rings is a film series based on the novel by J. R. R. Tolkien. *The Lord of the Rings* is widely regarded as one of the greatest and most influential film series ever made. It is among the highest-grossing film series of all time, with a cumulative world wide gross of $887,832,826 (imdb.com, 2020a). Each of the three films was critically acclaimed and won numerous prestigious film awards, including seventeen Academy Awards (imdb.com, 2020a). This makes the films very well known and influential to a large audience. Although the books do contain characters with dwarfism, the way they are portrayed in the film differs and once again they are deemed to be humorous. In her interview, Naomi spoke somewhat about the 'sport' of dwarf throwing, which involves a person with dwarfism being thrown across a room by someone of average stature purely for entertainment purposes. The 'sport' originated in Australia but gained popularity in various countries including the US and UK. However, it is now illegal in some countries, such as France, and in some US states, including Florida and New York. Although not mentioned in the book, the fact that this part was added to the film relates to Haberer, (2010) suggestion that people with dwarfism are used in movies mostly for novelty purposes linked to their stature. The fact that 'dwarf throwing' is mentioned in the film reinforces the connection between people with dwarfism and an action which is seen as not only humorous but also objectifies them. A person with dwarfism being used as something to be thrown, like a ball, is to be dehumanised (Van Etten, 1988). Humiliation is the attempt to lower someone below the status of a human being and as a person with dignity through improper attitude or treatment (Neuhauser, 2011: 22). Being treated like an object, as in the case of dwarf throwing, is an attempt to rid someone of their human status. Joan and Steve also point out how they think people with dwarfism are portrayed as something humorous and as an object:

How do you think dwarfs are stereotyped within the media? (Erin)
There are two ways [interrupted] (Joan)
Figures of comedy (Steve)
Yeah, figures of comedy as in circus clowns and things. There is a campaign on at the moment for The Range [a British home furnishing store]. Have you seen the advert? (Joan)
Yes (Erin)
They are using lots of dwarfs as gnomes. The gnomes were falling into the pools and making fools of themselves (Joan)

The characters with dwarfism are again used for mockery. The portrayal of disabled people in advertising encourages negative representations of them (Barnes and Mercer, 2010). Using dwarfs to play the role of the gnomes reinforces the connection between the two. In the case of using people with dwarfism as gnomes, the small figurines people put in the bottom of their garden, the portrayal makes them an object that can be used for display purposes. Garden gnomes are derived from the stone dwarf figures that were once popular in European gardens (Jagiełło-Kołaczyk, 2009). Gnomes, or stone dwarf figurines, were used as a status symbol, to reflect the court dwarfs kept by European royalty. Although garden gnomes are no longer used as status symbols, but rather just ornamental garden decorations, they are reflective of representations of people with dwarfism in less enlightened times. Kayleigh further talks about how people with dwarfism are seen as commodities and used as sources of amusement:

> *... We're also shown as something you can buy ... It was interesting with that incident at the Super Bowl [An Annual American Football Tournament], if you go onto the Little People's Association [An American association for people with dwarfism] website. One of the comedians stood up [stop] they had hired all these people of short stature to do impressions of famous people, so you were getting all these mini impressions of famous people, and the comedian stood up and said, 'Midgets are great, everybody should have one'. It's like they are something that you would buy, like they are something that you would keep because they are funny and entertaining (Kayleigh).*

Hiring someone out on the premise that their impairment can be mocked is an attempt to humiliate. Someone can feel humiliated without in fact being humiliated (Neuhauser, 2011). Imagine watching a show where there is someone who shares the same identity as you and everyone is laughing at that person's identity. How would you feel? The representation of people with dwarfism as commodities, which people can own suggests that people with dwarfism are viewed as subhuman. Suggesting that dwarfs can be kept for the amusement of others is not so different from owning a garden gnome. What Kayleigh talks about would reflect some of the historical representations of people with dwarfism, where they were often kept as pets, given as gifts or traded in European courts (Garland-Thomson, 1996). The concept of human dignity is meant to distinguish human beings from other creatures, notably animals (Kaufmann, et al., 2011). To be kept as a pet or to be owned, which subsequently puts people with dwarfism on par with a pet, impacts their dignity. Furthermore, Derkesen, (2020) points out that court dwarfs were always pictured with their 'owners' which indicated that they were not autonomous human beings. A person lacking dignity is associated with powerlessness (Kaufmann, et al., 2011). This indicates that they were humiliated as they had limited self-dignity.

What is problematic on this occasion is that there were dwarf entertainers promoting this sort of attitude by allowing themselves to be mocked. The Super Bowl is a very popular American sports event. For example, the 2015 Superbowl was watched by 114.4 million people, making it the most watched show in American television history (Patra, 2014). Dwarf entertainers provide the consent for others to hold disablist beliefs about people with dwarfism. If dwarf entertainers are seen consenting to being ridiculed, then it allows other members of the public to think that people with dwarfism are acceptable to mock. A few dwarf entertainers adhering to disablist representations limiting the agency other people with dwarfism have over their bodies. Joanne points out that people seem to be unaware of the offence caused through perpetuating stereotypes of dwarfism:

> *I think part of the problem is that people in the media are not aware of the offence they produce with perpetuating dwarf stereotypes and have yet to catch-up or be towed in line that dwarfism is an -ism—just like racism, disablism, sexism. I've had editors say to me you can't censor words when I was trying to explain that the term 'midget' is an equally offensive term like 'nigger' to a black person or 'faggot' to a gay person. Yet neither of those words would make the air with ease that the term 'midget' does across mainstream channels. My argument falls on deaf ears and the stereotypes are perpetuated (Joanne).*

There is a shared feeling amongst people with dwarfism that other minority groups, including other impairment groups are not treated in the same way that they are in the media. For example, it would not be seen as acceptable to comment on owning someone who is visually impaired. Adelson, (2005a) points out that political correctness in relation to dwarfism is practically nonexistent. As apparent in Joanne's quote as well as some of the others, the term 'midget' is used despite it being an offensive term. It is often pointed out that, 'using the term "midget" towards a dwarf is the same as calling a person of African descent a "n" (word)' (Kruse, 2002: 176). Although both terms are offensive, only one is deemed unacceptable. Although banning the N-word from use in the media does not eradicate racism, it does convey the message that it will not be tolerated; however, disablism in relation to dwarfism is still permitted. Joanne has clearly made an attempt to educate officials in the media who have denied that using terms such as 'midget' is offensive. This creates a power imbalance and allows the non-disabled person control over how dwarfism is represented. Naomi talks about a similar situation, but states that it takes more people to influence change:

> *It was a term [midget] that kept getting used again and again, I was objecting to several programmes on television and the advertising standards agency, and they just said it was a term that's not offensive.*

> *We know it is, but we as a group had not communicated that effectively to the wider world so it needed some sort of authority, so what I decided to do was I went and said in the [name of dwarf organisation] was can we pass a resolution guys that we as a group are definitely not happy with being called midget, and it was passed without exception. It was unanimous. Every hand in the room shot up and said we agree; we as a group of people do not want to be called this word. It's now disappearing. It's not disappeared but it's going ... but I do wish it had been done about 20 years ago ... (Naomi).*

Naomi is a member of an association for people with dwarfism and demonstrated an active involvement in trying to change how people with dwarfism are treated, including within the media. Naomi now thinks that due to the collaborative opinions of people with dwarfism the term 'midget' is now being used less within the media, but that this change is relatively new, especially in comparison to other minority groups.

5.3.1 A little positivity

As shown for centuries dwarfism, has been represented as a form of amusement, often in a way that constructs them as subhuman. However, with pushes for disability equality, including the Equality Act (2010) and American's with Disabilities Act (1990), more people with dwarfism have the opportunity to work in other occupations. Furthermore, those who do wish to work in the entertainment industry are striving for more positive roles, which emphasise their talents rather than their size. For example, the Emmy-award winning actor Peter Dinklage refuses to play roles that demean his dwarfism. In some cases, there is some indication of more positive representations of people with dwarfism within a few television programmes and films, including an actress with dwarfism who starred in Eastenders, a popular British soap opera:

> *There are some and I think that's good. There is a little person in Eastenders ..., We do need more in more serious roles that would be a good thing ... I think it would make the public see us in a different light and they would take us more seriously (Joan and Steve).*

> *There was that woman in Eastenders and there is Ellie Simmonds the swimmer [won several medals, including gold, at both the Beijing and London Paralympics]. I don't think there are many others you can admire because ones in show business are usually playing on the stereotype which makes it worse for us ... Ellie showed that she is a good swimmer and the woman in Eastenders was just a normal character. She didn't run around and make a fool of herself like others have (Amanda).*

An actor with dwarfism playing the role of a more 'normal' character or taking on a more 'serious role' helps to break away the connection between dwarfism and ridicule or as something from mythology. To see someone with dwarfism acting in a non-derogatory way shows that representations may slowly be improving and that this can help to change how they are perceived. It can help to disconnect the relation between having dwarfism and automatically being seen as someone to be laughed at. In Amanda's case, the actors with dwarfism who do not construct dwarfism as something to laugh at are the ones who she admires. However, Meeuf, (2014) claims that the celebration of Peter Dinklage's success ignores the wider problem of how people with dwarfism are represented within the entertainment industry. Amanda further points out actors with dwarfism who humiliate themselves do not help how society views and treats people with dwarfism and thus are hard to admire:

> *I don't think there are many others [people with dwarfism] you can admire because ones in show business are usually playing on the stereotype which makes it worse for us. How can you admire someone who is making a complete arse of themselves and showing dwarfism as something funny and ok to make fun of? (Amanda).*

Amanda, like the majority of participants, spoke about receiving a lot of unwanted attention within society, much of which she felt was influenced by cultural representations of dwarfism. Amanda clearly finds it hard to admire someone who can influence how she is treated within society, as according to her they socially construct dwarfism as humorous. Oliver, (1990) suggests that dominant cultural images of disabled people, which in this case are people with dwarfism who are represented as humorous, are unhelpful in providing role models and add to the prejudice disabled people encounter in society.

It is apparent that people with dwarfism consider cultural representations of dwarfism to be constructed as something that can be ridiculed as it is deemed humorous. This indicates that dwarfism is socially constructed as something humorous, and this is connected to their visible bodily difference, most notably their small stature. 'Characters with dwarfism that are popularised on television, in films and children's games present people with dwarfism as creatures in caves, exotic "sidekicks", or persons with special or magical abilities' (Ablon, 1990: 885). There is a lack of roles which reflect a more realistic portrayal of dwarfism.

The majority of participants pointed out that people with dwarfism are used as commodities, apparent in mythology and were prominent in the Victorian freak shows and that these representations are still prevalent today within the media. 'Among other "disabilities" dwarfism has a unique and ambiguous history with roots in mythology, the commodification of anomalous bodies through enfreakment and the pathologising of bodily differences' (Kruse, 2003: 496). These representations were commented to have a strong presence throughout history and to the present day. These representations differ from the range of social complexities and experiences that make up the lives of people with dwarfism.

There is some indication that people with dwarfism are beginning to be given more mainstream and serious roles within films and on television shows, indicating that representations of dwarfism may be changing and focusing less on dwarfism as something humorous or mystic. I now want to move on and explore how particular representations can affect people with dwarfism within public spaces.

5.4 The social consequences of cultural representations

Cultural images and myths are a contributing factor to disabled people's discrimination within society (Barnes, 1991b; Shakespeare, 1994; Thomas, 2004). Wendell, (1996) suggests that culture has an effect in constructing a misleading representation of disabled people. Barnes and Mercer, (2010) suggest that the effects that the media has on how disabled people are treated within society is limited. Numerous works that has explored how people with dwarfism have been culturally represented (Adelson, 2005b; Brown, 2020; Derksen, 2020; Mock, 2020; Solevag, 2020; Tyrrell, 2020; Watson, 2020) but limited engagement with the social implications of these representations. Whilst people with dwarfism are prominent in the media, the implications have so far gone unnoticed within wider society.

In relation to the cultural representations of disability, theories of how the media influences people's perception and attitudes, or 'media effects', can aid in understanding how the cultural representations of dwarfism can influence how other people view and treat those with dwarfism. The agenda-setting theory asserts that people's understanding of social reality is copied from the media (Shaw, 1979). It is assumed that mass media has a strong, long-term effect on audiences, based on a constant stream of messages that is presented. Thus, it is more of an accumulation of a particular issue that will reinforce people's ideas. For example, as noted by Garland-Thomson, (1997), Ablon, (1990) and Adelson, (2005b) people with dwarfism have a long history of being portrayed as oddities and thus are likely to be viewed this way by other members of the public. The constant representation of dwarfism as an oddity may influence others to perceive dwarfism in the same way. Gerbner and Gross, (1974) suggest that entertainment television shapes people's perceptions of reality. If dwarfism is constantly presented in a particular way, over time some people's views and attitudes towards dwarfism, and subsequently the way they interact with them, are likely to be influenced by them.

Cultural images and myths are a contributing factor to disabled people's discrimination within society (Barnes, 1991; Hevey, 1992; Shakespeare, 1994; Thomas, 2004). Focusing on cultural stereotypes and personal beliefs

Heider, et al., (2013) argue that people's perceptions of people with dwarfism include weird, incapable and childlike and that they are perceived as objects of entertainment. These resonate with perceptions explored in the previous section. The cultural representations of people with dwarfism can have an effect on how other members of the public perceive and interact with them, basing them on how they are portrayed within popular culture, including mass media. When people lack first-hand knowledge of an issue, they frequently turn to the media for information (Barnes, 1991b). The media provides easy access to gaining an insight about something but can also have the power to provide the wrong impression. Representation of dwarfism has implications for how people with dwarfism are perceived and treated within society, as Joanne points out:

Whether it is as a mystical figure, a freak or somebody to be mocked and a person has to be pretty naive to think that this portrayal does not have an effect on the rest of the dwarf community. It does. It gives people on the street permission to treat us the way they see dwarfs on TV/Film who have consented to being treated a particular way (Joanne).

Although people with dwarfism, within the media have consented to being mocked because of their short stature, this can unfortunately encourage society to treat people with dwarfism in the same way. However, people with dwarfism in society have not given their consent to be treated as a humorous spectacle, as shown in the previous section. This opens up all kinds of ethical debates concerning the career choices of the minority. Jade further argues that representations affect how people expect her to respond to people perceiving her as funny because she has dwarfism:

They [people with dwarfism in entertainment] were either funny or scary and that's how people reacted towards me constantly, I was either funny or scary. Still some of that happens today; people expect you to be up laughing and joking all the time and if you are not it's because you are not a nice person or because you have a problem accepting your own shortness (Jade).

Jade makes a link between how people with dwarfism are portrayed and thus how she is expected to behave in society. Shakespeare, et al. (2007) suggest that people with dwarfism are assumed to have a particular personality trait by other members of the public. In this case, it is humorous, and if Jade is not laughing, then she is viewed as unpleasant and that she cannot accept her own shortness which people connect with humour, rather than that she does not want to use her height as a source of amusement for others. A person with dwarfism who does not act like the stereotypical dwarfs within the media create an incongruous encounter and challenge heightist assumptions. 'Other members of the public tend to see dwarfs as figures of fun' (Shakespeare, et al., 2010: 30). It is as if people assume that all people with dwarfism will be happy to amuse others. This can affect how they are perceived, which Michelle further points out:

> *... Sometimes you have these dwarf throwing parties and I don't like things like that ... I think it puts us in a bad light and a lot of us are well educated, but Joe public will think that is all we can do (Michelle).*

According to Michelle, misrepresenting people with dwarfism can distort the fact that they lead ordinary lives, and instead she believes that many members of the public will connect people like her with the mis-representations. Our self-respect is highly dependent on the social role played by those groups we belong to (Neuhauser, 2011). This is why it is important to consider how people with dwarfism are culturally re-presented, as the career choices of some dwarfs in the entertainment industry can impact upon the self-respect of people with dwarfism in general. Often people assume that derogatory entertainment is what people with dwarfism have to do for a living, as they are deemed in-capable of regular employment. This conception is as disablist as it is racist to think that certain ethnic minorities only work in particular occupations. Michelle mentions dwarf throwing, which several other participants also spoke about, and sees it as something which is de-grading and which does not give people with dwarfism a good image. As well as other events, dwarf throwing is featured in numerous films, in-cluding the 2013 film *The Wolf of Wall Street*[1]. People with dwarfism are concerned that dwarf throwing will encourage people to pick them up on the street and throw them (Van Etten, 1988). Ivy explains how dwarf throwing made her apprehensive about how people would treat her sons who both have dwarfism:

> *Have you experienced any times when these sorts of stereotypes like the humorous person have been directed at you? (Erin)*
> *People laugh at me and take the Mickey ... I did get concerned when there was dwarf throwing, and I have got two sons and when they were younger it only takes for somebody to come along and pick them up and treat it not just as a game, luckily that never happened. I have only been abused in taking the Mickey such as name-calling and laughing (Ivy).*

Although the incident never occurred, Ivy shows that she was worried about how dwarf throwing could have affected her sons, and this could be related to the fact that she points out that other representations of dwarfism have affected her in the past. The anxiety Ivy experiences in public is a form of psycho-emotional disablism. Naomi further sug-gests that dwarf throwing affects how people interact with people with dwarfism:

> *I think Danny Baker [British writer, journalist and radio DJ] did not help us at all. It was Danny Baker that brought dwarf tossing over here. It appeared on some shows including the Chris Tarrant production. They didn't condemn it; they just said this is what happens, let's go and look at this funny clip of this short person being chucked into a crash mat and all the audience laughs. But that gets it into the social conscience that this is acceptable. Remember how many short people there are, there are very few of us. If you have got a handful of individuals making absolute pillocks of themselves, then we have to suffer the consequences … I don't want to be manually handled (Naomi).*

Naomi mentioned in her interview that on a night out one man picked her up without her consent, indicating to her that certain members of the public do think it is acceptable to pick up people with dwarfism. Adelson, (2005b) points out that dwarf tossing encouraged some people to pick up people with dwarfism and swing them about. Again, people with dwarfism are treated like an object as opposed to a person. The concept of social dignity can be seen as an argument for group rights to equal treatment. This means that the social implications that cultural representations of dwarfism have on the dignity of people with dwarfism within society needs more consideration. If a particular representation impacts their equal treatment in society, then it needs to be questioned if it is morally right to allow that representation to exist, especially when it is exposed to a large audience.

The rarity of dwarfism provides the media, which is broadcasted to a large audience, to have more influence in how dwarfism is perceived in society. Joanne further discusses how people with dwarfism are shown as something which can be picked up, which can affect how people with dwarfism act within public spaces:

> *… it's permissible to pick up a RG [restricted growth, another term for a person with dwarfism] without consent because certain quarters of the media objectify dwarfs. We like to play things to certain sections of the general public, something to have a laugh about with their mates either walking down the street or in a bar. I can't help think the Johnny Depp [famous Hollywood actor] episode of* Life's Too Short *[comedy sitcom about a person with dwarfism] where he gets Warwick [Davies] to stand in a toilet, has put back what little respect and equality we've achieved over the last couple of years, back a decade or two, or actually reinforced the stereotype that we are a 'thing' to play with. I was also disappointed that such a respected actor would participate in such a sketch—even if both men are playing parodies of themselves. Not everyone is intelligent enough or aware enough to discern this (Joanne).*

The programme Joanne talks about, which has also been mentioned earlier, came out in the UK in 2012, making it a very modern show which continues to perpetuate people with dwarfism as something which can be picked up and ridiculed. To be stuck in a toilet by an average-sized actor, indicates a lack of power which permits others to treat them in an inferior manner. Strangely, the actor Wareick Davis is also a patron of Little People UK (LPUK), which claims to promote equality for people with dwarfism. However, Warwick often remains silent when concerns are raised about particular representations of dwarfism when promoted by dwarf entertainers. Joanne mentions that Johnny Depp, a famous Hollywood actor, appears in the programme that will increase the show's popularity (Sancho, 2003). Attracting a large audience will increase the show's influence across society, increasing the likelihood of people responding to people with dwarfism in society in the same way. There will be some members of society who are led to believe that people with dwarfism are acceptable to ridicule. Jade further backs up what Joanne claims by talking about a past experience:

> *I used to be called Bridget the midget. When I was growing up a song came out called 'Bridget the Midget', and of course everyone at school would call me Bridget for ages. It wasn't really bullying; it was just them associating, because that was the first time on television that they had seen somebody tiny. I can't remember whether it was just a scaled down version of somebody or a short person was actually used in the video. It was on* Top of the Pops *[British music show] and really popular. From then on, it became acceptable to use that term for then onwards because it had been seen on the television and that (Jade).*

Jade was automatically associated with 'Bridget the Midget' as they both shared something in common which not many people in society will. The fact that the name contains the word 'midget' can be seen as offensive as every participant interviewed recalled finding that name very offensive and one which they would never use to refer to their dwarfism. 'Midget' derives from the word 'midge' meaning sandfly or gnat, which is dehumanising. It was popularised within the freak shows, where people with dwarfism were exploited. Pritchard, (2019) argues that the term is a form of hate speech, but unlike other forms of hate speech, it is used freely within the media. Nearly all twenty-two participants recalled being called a midget by other members of the public, and, in all cases, the name was used to offend. As noted in the previous section, there is work which is being done to remove the word midget from the media, although this has been met with some difficulties. Joanne further points out that name-calling in society is encouraged by the use of certain names in the media:

> *I think the general public attitude about dwarfs reflects the behaviour that is tolerated in the media. It's permissible to call a RG [Restricted Growth] person a midget … (Joanne).*

Allowing the name midget to be used in the media can encourage its acceptance as a word that can be used towards people with dwarfism as well as increasing its popularity.

5.4.1 Ethical considerations of the choices of a few

Representations of dwarfism are constructed by the average-sized person; however, it is the dwarf entertainers who aid in keeping the problem alive through their consent to perform. The neoliberal belief that everyone needs to work overrides the ethical implications that this form of employment has on the group's collective dignity. 'If humiliation is directed against a collectively shared part of identity, the whole group is humiliated and not only the violated individual' (Neuhauser, 2011: 27). This is why ethical consideration is required when thinking about the rights of those wanting to partake in derogatory entertainment. They may have free choice to humiliate themselves, however, the rest of the group is also humiliated. This humiliation does not just occur within a person's psyche, but also through the actions of others, such as name-calling. Nearly half the participants blamed people with dwarfism in the entertainment business for the unwanted attention they received from other members of the public:

> *Because somebody on television who is a little person is being stupid or funny or whatever, then they naturally assume that everybody who is like that is going to be like that (Amy).*

The perception that all people with dwarfism act in a stupid or funny way can encourage the same audience perception to people with dwarfism in society:

> *I don't think it is very good, and I kind of think why are they humiliating themselves in that role. It just makes me think that the next day when I am walking down the street someone sees a little person like me what are they going to be thinking? (Alison).*

Being perceived in the same way as a dwarf entertainer, who has consented to being ridiculed, creates an ethical dilemma where people with dwarfism who do not consent to be ridiculed to nonetheless be treated in a derogatory manner within society:

> *The thing that gets me is that some of the small people like that guy [Verne Troyer, a dwarf actor] in Austin Powers, I would like to beat that guy up because he can get shit loads of money for it but we have to live with the shit that comes from it (Anne).*

The actor Ann is referring to is Verne Troyer who appeared as the character 'Mini-Me' in two out of the three Austin Powers movies[2]. Mini-Me was first introduced as a clone of Austin Power's arch nemesis Dr Evil. He is described as an exact clone of Dr Evil except one-eight his size. Along with his name, the description of him automatically places emphasis upon his stature. In early cinema, dwarfs often fulfiled the role of children or played diminutive mimics of average-sized characters (Adelson, 2005a). Mini-Me's character is almost a combination of these two roles. Whilst he does not play the role of a child, he is infantilised throughout the film, and, as shown, does not have his own personality, but that of Dr Evil's. Throughout the two films Mini-Me (or more specifically his height) is used as a comedic crutch. Backstrom, (2012) suggests that Verne Troyer's 'Mini-Me' is seen as a negative representation of dwarfism as his dwarfism is mocked for humour. What is most problematic is that his name has become synonymous with dwarfism and has added to the numerous derogatory names that people with dwarfism are called:

> *The Austin Powers films came out and there were a couple of times in clubs when guys would call me 'Mini-Me' or 'Mrs Mini-Me' (Jennifer).*

A connection is made between the character with dwarfism and someone with dwarfism in society. It reduces Jennifer to one identity, which is associated with mockery, which influences how people interact with people with dwarfism, including verbal abuse. It is as if they are given free reign to mock people with dwarfism because the media can often be used as a device to judge what is permissible behaviour. For example, if a term is deemed offensive it is banned from the media. Equally, if a scene in a film is later deemed inappropriate it is cut from the film. However, in relation to dwarfism, there seems to be no ethical cut off point. As apparent by the character's name that the focus was once again upon their height, which Myraar further points out is a funny character:

> *Everywhere I go they just say, 'that's a midget' or 'that is a Mini-Me'. It is all those characters and they are all quite funny characters (Myraar).*

For Myraar saying 'that is a Mini-Me' shows that her dwarfism is connected to a film character, and subsequently she is not seen as a person with dwarfism but a 'Mini-Me', reducing her identity to one derogatory representation. This character presents a false representation of dwarfism, but for some people in society, seems to be their only point of reference for people with dwarfism. Referring to her as 'a Mini-Me' shows that Myraar is not a person with dwarfism in a conventional sense, but a 'Mini-Me' who is, as Myraar points out, portrayed as 'funny' which again connects dwarfism with being funny or unusual. The character overrides Myraar's true identity and instead constructs her as an amusing being. Amanda also mentions names she's been called which relate to characters with dwarfism:

I have been called 'Mini-Me' and been asked where Snow White is. It happens quite often, I think people are just trying to show off to their friends. They think because a dwarf in film or on TV is ok with it, we must all be ok with it and enjoy people making fun out of our height (Amanda).

When dwarf entertainers allow themselves to be ridiculed on television or in a film, it encourages other members of the public to make fun of people with dwarfism. Laughter is a social phenomenon (Billig, 2005). It can help to build social relations by acknowledging similarities within social groups. Having a sense of humour is deemed a good social trait and, therefore, using a person with dwarfism as a comedic prop to encourage others to deem you humorous can aid in building social bonds. This may be why some people with dwarfism choose to allow people to laugh at them, as it may be a way for them to become part of a social group. However, allowing themselves to be laughed at actually places them within a inferior position within society. Heider, et al. (2013) suggest that how some people with dwarfism capitalise on their height in the entertainment industry creates a cultural perception of dwarfism as an object of amusement and entertainment.

One of the main representations to be mentioned was *Snow White and the Seven Dwarfs*, which is not only a popular fairy tale, but also an animated movie created by Disney, a highly popular film company aimed pre-dominantly at children. Giroux and Pollock, (2010) argue that Disney is a multimillion dollar global corporation which has a significant influence over popular culture. Disney's animated version of Snow White and the Seven Dwarfs was Disney's first film, made in 1937, and remains one of its most popular films, attracting a wide audience. Adelson, (2005b) points out that if asked to recall a film that features characters with dwarfism, Snow White and the Seven Dwarfs is the most popular answer. As well as the animated film, there are also regular theatre productions of the story in the form of pantomimes, making them a very well-known set of characters. Naomi and Lydia further point out how Snow White is used by other members of the public to mock them:

I got a few 'Heigh Hos' whistled at me in the street … (Naomi).

… the Snow White and the Seven Dwarfs stereotype. When I was in Blackpool a few years ago to see a friend who was in Snow White and the Seven Dwarfs, *we went out for a meal and people started singing behind us 'Heigh Ho' (Lydia).*

The song Naomi and Lydia are referring to is a well-known song which the seven dwarfs sing in Disney's animated version of *Snow White and the Seven Dwarfs*. Disney is famous for creating animated musicals and many of the songs are very well known within society. The experiences demonstrate that some other members of public associate Lydia and Naomi with the popular fairy tale and this affected how both were then treated. Ivy further mentions and how it can have an effect on how children interact with people with dwarfism:

> *Snow White and the Seven Dwarfs, they always play a comic part really and it's a thing that makes people laugh. I mean it's difficult for parents to take their children to see* Snow White and the Seven Dwarfs *and encourage them to laugh and then when they come out the theatre somebody like me walks along and they tell them not to laugh. It must be very confusing for that to happen to a child (Ivy).*

In Disney's animated version of the fairy tale, the seven dwarfs are used for comedic purposes. For example, they are often seen acting silly, tripping over themselves and in several scenes are laughed at by Snow White. Watson, (2020) suggests that 'Snow White and the Seven Dwarfs teaches the audience that people with dwarfism are funny looking and childlike and that it is okay to laugh at them'. Ivy believes that the representation of dwarfs in Snow White affects how people, especially children, react to people with dwarfism in society. Shakespeare (1994: 2) points out that 'as children grow up, they learn about disabled people through books, films and legends which they encounter', and so real disabled people are understood in terms of fictional stereotypes. A person with dwarfism is easily recognisable, and, if a child has no other point of reference to a person with dwarfism, then their perception is likely to be shaped by the person with dwarfism on stage. Sofia also explains how representations of dwarfism can distort the realities of living with dwarfism:

> *It is like we are not supposed to do normal things, or you know we are just shown as an entertainer for them to look at. I think for them they don't see us doing normal things; as far as they know we are there for entertainment like a wrestler or someone in a carnival. It is impossible for them to think that we can have a normal life, you know that kind of thing. Obviously, from the moment you go out, you get looks, you get abuse, you get called names and obviously it is not good ... I just think people take the piss out of us because of the way we entertain people ... they just take the piss out of you because you are a little person (Sofia).*

Unwanted social attention, including name-calling, is apparent when people with dwarfism are in public spaces and these, according to Sofia, are influenced by representations of dwarfism. Arial and Lydia talk about how some members of the public connect people with dwarfism to the circus:

> *I think the older people still associate us with the circus, and when they see me they think there is a circus nearby (Arial).*

I remember as a child my Mum and Dad were fans of the circus association because my Dad was a clown in a circus and an old lady would say there is a circus in town, that type of thing. Again, paint brushing you because all dwarfs are clowns. (Lydia).

Four participants, including Aerial and Lydia, felt that their presence indicated to other members of the public that there must be a circus in their area. In the previous section of the chapter, it was pointed out that part of the historical representations of dwarfism are linked to the circus, which may be why in both cases they think that the older generation associates them more with the circus. Lydia's parents both had dwarfism and were a part of the circus, but Lydia criticises the assumption that all dwarfs must be circus clowns, which again is something to laugh at. Just as it is racist to assume that particular ethic minorities work in particular occupations, it is disablist to assume that people with dwarfism work in the circus. Assuming that people with dwarfism work in a circus reduces them to a humorous spectacle. A number of other participants also think that representations of dwarfs, including past representations, will leave people mocking them in the same way dwarfs are mocked within the media:

They had this absolutely awful sketch [Little and Large; *a popular double act famous throughout the 1980s*]. *I would have been about 10. It was prime time television on BBC [Popular UK television channel] so lots would have been watching. They got the tallest man in Britain and the shortest man in Britain, and the shortest man of Britain running in and out of the tallest man's legs … That was BBC; it wasn't some peculiar Sky channel [Sky—A multi-channel service] that was something millions of people would have been watching … The humour wasn't at the individual it was at his stature and it means that when the rest of us have to go for a job interview, what image is going to be in that interviewers head as you are walking through the door? It's going to be what they saw on television, … It's like people always think we are happy being the butt of the joke. He wasn't making the joke, he was the butt of it (Naomi).*

Although shown over thirty years ago, the sketch seems to have stuck with Naomi and is still relevant to her today. The scene Naomi describes can be associated with the Victorian freak shows where dwarfs and giants often performed together in order to exaggerate their height (Garland-Thomson, 1996). This demonstrates that the focus was upon the dwarf's stature and through exaggerating his height further draws focus upon it. In this scenario, the tall man is used as a prop not only to exaggerate how short the dwarf is, but also for the dwarf to ridicule himself by running in between the legs of the tall man. Not only standing there but running around and showing how his shortness can create a humorous situation, and this encourages people with dwarfism to be seen as the butt of the joke, especially due to the high exposure of the media. This Naomi thinks will impact the employment opportunities for people with dwarfism:

> ... *The humour wasn't at the individual, it was at his stature and it means that when the rest of us have to go for a job interview, what image is going to be in that interviewer's head as you are walking through the door? It's going to be what they saw on television... It's like people always think we are happy being the butt of the joke. He wasn't making the joke, he was the butt of it (Naomi).*

Events and shows which focus on and ridicule a person with dwarfism affects people's perception of dwarfism, which in turn causes difficulties for them within society, such as obtaining employment (Van Etten, 1988). As the entertainer with dwarfism was making fun of his size, Naomi also thinks it will give people reason to believe that all people with dwarfism are happy with their short stature being an object of ridicule. This can impact how potential employers perceive people with dwarfism. Being discriminated against in a job because of preconceived ideas of dwarfism, based on dwarf entertainment, impacts the self-respect of others. Although the Equality Act (2010) aims to reduce discriminatory barriers to employment, it is easy for employers to covertly discriminate against people with dwarfism based on their perceptions of them. Lawyer Paul Steven Miller, for example, a person with dwarfism, reflects upon how he struggled to gain employment, with one law firm noting their reason for rejecting him was that their clients would think that they were running a 'circus freak show' (Adelson, 2005a). A lawyer with dwarfism creates an incongruous encounter. A lawyer is a professional with a strong educational background, which juxtaposes representations of dwarfism in the media. German lawyer Silke Schönfleisch-Backofen, who has dwarfism, successfully sued a man after he started laughing and singing 'Heigh Ho' at her in court (Reuters, 2012). Lydia goes on and makes a distinction between the different ways of using humour and how it can affect people with dwarfism:

> *Depends on how it's being portrayed in a humorous way. If it's a humorous way as in any other comedian, actor or actress as being in a humorous way then that's fine. If it is a humorous way as in degrading or belittling that person, I would be concerned how it would affect other dwarfs either seeing it or people watching it. They could possibly paint us all with the same brush. If they see one dwarf being stupid some people may assume we all act stupid and that it's ok to be that degrading to people that they come across (Lydia).*

There is a difference between being laughed '*at*' and laughed '*with*'. The former is degrading as it constructs the person being laughed at as inferior. Reid, et al. (2006) examine how stand-up comedy in the US perpetuates negative attitudes towards disabled people but argue that 'disability humour' can promote a positive identity for disabled people. Haller and Ralph, (2003) suggest that disability humour that challenges ableist assumptions and disability stereotypes helps to challenge attitudes towards disability. Kayleigh further discusses how different representations have affected her:

> *I am very aware that when a film comes out if there is a person in that being portrayed negatively. I will get that screamed at me down the street. What I find fascinating is for example is 'Time Bandits' …That has never been used towards me where as 'Mini-me' has, and if you analyse the film, the roles of the little people within those films are vastly different. One is the butt of jokes and the other is the protagonist, and I think it is really interesting that roles where a little person is empowered have never been used to attack me (Kayleigh).*

The fact that Kayleigh points out those names are 'screamed' at her in the street suggests that the way representations of people with dwarfism are used towards her are often used in a threatening manner. Kayleigh, an actress who pointed out in her interview that she never takes on roles which are degrading to her dwarfism, especially since they could have an effect on her and her sisters who both share the same type of dwarfism as her. Kayleigh considers some representations of dwarfism in films to have more of a negative effect than others. The more negative representations are often where the character is someone to be laughed at, such as Mini-Me. This demonstrates that more positive representations of people with dwarfism, which were partly discussed in the first section, would help to change society's attitudes towards them.

As well as being deemed humorous, people with dwarfism are also constructed as mythical. Haberer, (2010) suggests that the media presents dwarfism as something abnormal and mythical. Furthermore, an unusual body that goes beyond what is considered normal, in this case body size, goes into the realm of mythical (Semonin, 1996). In mythology, dwarfs are depicted alongside elves, leprechauns, imps, dragons and unicorns. This makes them seem mythical and unreal, as opposed to actual disabled people. Dwarfs in mythology are understood to be men with long beards, wearing a Viking's helmet, and often carrying an axe, and the presence of any females with dwarfism is practically nonexistent (see for example Tolkien's *Lord of the Rings Trilogy*). A number of these films are based on historical novels and fairy tales. Being perceived as mythical can result in various reactions and unwanted encounters, including being touched inappropriately:

> *I have had people touch me for good luck because they think I am a leprechaun (Lydia).*

In chapter 2, it was discussed that the cultural rules of engagement, such as not saying something inappropriate, are often ignored by other members of the public when they are interacting with people with dwarfism. In these instances, again the cultural rules of engagement have been ignored, which is not touching someone, and it can be argued that they have been affected by how some cultures perceive dwarfism. Massie and Mayer, (2014) argue that people with dwarfism are most prominent in medieval imagery, which is often associated with mythology. Lydia points out that the people who touched her thought she was a leprechaun, a fairy tale creature that is linked to mythology and Irish folklore, as opposed to a disabled person. A connection between dwarfism and mythology arouses fascination from other members of the public, often causing people to believe that people with the impairment are not fully human (Goffman, 1963). This indicates that in some communities dwarfism is connected more with fiction rather than being seen as an impairment. Mock, (2020) representations of mythical dwarfs combine physical attributes of dwarfism and longstanding folk motifs, which blur the boundary between fiction and disability. The people touching Lydia did not see a person with a physical impairment, but rather a mythical being that they would have come across in cultural folktales. Being touched can provoke psycho-emotional disablism:

> *I had one really bad incident in London. It was awful. I got surrounded by Gypsies [sic] who were all trying to touch me for good luck. Very threatening situation and I was so distraught by it (Kayleigh).*

> *There are people in other cultures where they think you are very lucky, they think you are a lucky charm. I was in Llandudno [seaside town in North Wales] only last year and a huge Irish family appeared where they all wanted to touch me and my daughter. There were one or two of them, and they called the family over, and they all wanted to touch us because we were lucky charms. They were very polite about it saying, 'do you mind if we touch you?' Well I am not going to say no and have a big argument with them all, because we were in the middle of Llandudno. Really we are not that lucky, I have never won the lottery, we are just short, not lucky (Jade).*

Although the people who touched Jade, Lydia and Kayleigh meant no harm, it indicates a situation that they had to comply with, especially since both Kayleigh and Jade mention that the people wanting to touch them were in groups and would have been bigger than them. This demonstrates an imbalance of power. However, Jade avoids resistance, as it could lead to an unwanted interaction. Not complying with the ableist perception of dwarfism will result in an incongruous encounter, which constructs the person with dwarfism, not as a happy, bringer of good fortune, but rather a regular person, who like anyone else does not want to be touched by strangers. As in the case of Kayleigh, the situation is a form of psycho-emotional disablism.

Whilst in some cultures people with dwarfism are seen as a good omen, in others they may be perceived differently:

> *I would say I experience more in my country where dwarf is not recognised at all. It is bad luck, and people would cross the road when I was walking, and they would say to my face how bad luck I am and how it is all because of bad karma and because of what I did in my last life (Myraar).*

Myraar comes from a country in Southeast Asia, where cultural beliefs about dwarfism differ. It is not uncommon for some religions to believe that having an impairment is the result of doing something bad in a past life. This constructs disabled people as bad because their impairment is a sign of punishment. Mock, (2020) argues that mythical representations of dwarfism often correlate dwarfism to wickedness. Being considered a bad omen affects how others interact with her, including actively avoiding her. This shows that she does not belong and is treated as an outcast. This demonstrates that in different cultures dwarfism is recognised differently, and that various recognitions of people with dwarfism cause unwanted attention within public spaces. These stigmatising actions are a form of psycho-emotional disablism. Lydia also points out how these representations can affect how people with dwarfism are treated in comparison to other disabled people:

> *It's ok to do dwarf throwing but they wouldn't do wheelchair throwing or blind persons throwing or CP [Cerebral Palsy] throwing. I have got a few friends who are disabled, and when I am out and about with them or if I observe them from a while ago, they're not singled out as much as somebody with dwarfism or any form of restricted growth are (Lydia).*

According to Lydia, how people with dwarfism are portrayed differs significantly from how other disabled people are and this leads to her receiving more unwanted attention in society than some of her disabled friends. As pointed out in chapter 3, participants felt that when they used a wheelchair or mobility scooter unwanted attention towards them did decrease. Thus, cultural representations of dwarfism could be a contributing factor to a hierarchy of impairments. As shown in the first section of this chapter, the way people with dwarfism are represented differs significantly from their real lives. They are not portrayed as typical disabled people, but rather as spectacles which can be used for entertainment purposes. As Kennedy, (2003) argues, other disabled people, such as wheelchair users, do not rent themselves out purely for entertainment purposes. Other impairments, such as cerebral palsy, do not have the same entertaining history as dwarfism, and whilst not exempt from humour, are usually represented as tragic and pitiful, which would make mocking them in the same way as dwarfism seem cruel. However, people with dwarfism are constructed as happy beings, who relish in lowbrow entertainment.

It is apparent that, when people with dwarfism access public spaces, attitudes towards them from other members of the public are often reflective of cultural representations of dwarfism. This indicates that the media can affect how some people perceive and subsequently treat people with dwarfism. Barnes and Mercer, (2010) suggest that the lives of disabled people are affected by the negative reactions from other members of the public. 'Because most members of the general public do not know any dwarfs personally, their impressions are formed by what they see in popular culture' (Adelson, 2005a: 10). In most cases, it seemed that other members of the public found it acceptable to mock people with dwarfism, often relating them to a character which was deemed to be humorous. The rarity and novelty of dwarfism means that it is impossible for people with dwarfism to avoid the unwanted attention from other members of the public (Shakespeare, et al., 2010). Due to dwarfism's rarity, the continuing humiliation of the impairment within the media has a profound effect on the dignity of all people with dwarfism. Therefore, people with dwarfism may avoid certain spaces in order to reduce the amount of unwanted attention they receive, which lessens the amount of psycho-emotional disablism they personally experience.

5.4.2 Avoidance of spaces

As already shown in the previous chapters, the spatial practices of people with dwarfism are influenced by representations of spaces. Avoiding spaces due to the way people react to people with dwarfism can be seen as a form of social exclusion, which affects their participation within society, such as pursuing leisure activities. These leisure activities can include going to the local cinema or theatre, especially if the person is aware that a film on show features a character with dwarfism:

> I remember a few years ago going to see Austin Powers because I liked the first one. When Mini-Me came on, I cringed and was dreading walking out at the end because people would associate me with him, and again he was just something you laughed at because he was small. I think since then I have always been careful about what film I have gone to see (Amanda).

> If there's a little person in a film, I wouldn't go and see it at the cinema. I wouldn't want people to be watching me watch that (Naomi).

Amanda is apprehensive about how people may connect her to the dwarf character in a film, especially since people are encouraged to laugh at the character with dwarfism, and thus she will avoid films if they are likely to produce this situation. It is likely that Amanda would be the only person with dwarfism at the cinema, which would single her out more. Similarly, Naomi will avoid watching any film with a character with dwarfism in it as she perceives that it will draw focus upon her, adding to the unwanted attention she already receives from other members of society. As pointed out, dwarfism is a rare impairment and thus seeing someone with dwarfism in the audience, as well as within the film will provoke attention. How the character with dwarfism is portrayed will be fresh in people's minds, and if the character is something to be ridiculed, it is likely to affect the person with dwarfism in the audience. Avoiding a film with a character with dwarfism in it can be seen as a strategy which minimises how much unwanted attention both Amanda and Naomi receive, although one which restricts their choice and movement within public spaces. Joanne further points out how a representation of dwarfism on the television can leave her apprehensive about how the representation can affect her:

> *The latest small person representation on TV is in Ricky Gervais'* Life's Too Short *leaves me in a conundrum. I worry that because Warwick [A British actor with dwarfism] is happy to get into a toilet because he thinks he's going to get £5000 for it, doesn't necessarily mean that a dwarf on a night out who is made to do the same because the offender has seen it on the show, thinks it hilarious, and that as a dwarf we would find it funny to participate in such behaviour. This situation might not happen, but I've been in situations where I have control taken away from me because an average-height person thought it was funny to lift me up and place me somewhere it would be impossible for me to get down. The knock-on effect of such antics does make you think twice before going to certain areas or doing certain things where you know you leave yourself vulnerable (Joanne).*

What Joanne demonstrates is that representations make her apprehensive about where she will go as past experiences demonstrate that people often act in an inappropriate way towards her. This is a form of psycho-emotional disablism, as Joanne feels anxious due to her perceived vulnerability. Her small body size makes it easier for people to treat her this way, including picking her up, and thus again the cultural rules of engagement, which have been discussed in previous chapters, are broken. Avoiding certain spaces where past representations have affected her, helps to minimise the chance of the latest representation doing the same.

Most people with dwarfism have encountered other people staring at them. Shakespeare, et al. (2010) found that 98% of their participants, who all had dwarfism, had experienced being stared out when out in public. In all interviews, participants spoke about being stared at but seven mentioned also being photographed, which can be seen as an extreme form of staring (Garland–Thomson, 2002). Being photographed can lead to the avoidance of areas, especially in certain spaces, such as those connected to representations of people with dwarfism, as Naomi talks about:

> *I never want to be next to a poster advertising* Snow White; *I never want to be beneath the sign saying* Snow White, *because I never want to be that photo opportunity for someone with a camera phone (Naomi).*

Naomi is anxious about being in spaces that contain representations of dwarfism in case it provokes unwanted attention. This anxiety may arise from past experiences, which as Naomi pointed out previously, involved references to Snow White, and thus Naomi employs her own strategy to try and avoid any recurrence. Naomi spoke about how one association for people with dwarfism has been working on eradicating photographs of people with dwarfism taken by other members of the public and placed on social networking sites such as Facebook. On these sites, the photographs are uploaded, and people are encouraged to leave abusive comments next to them. Naomi, being well aware of this incident, shows why she is careful upon where she goes and why she will especially avoid somewhere displaying a derogatory stereotype associated with dwarfism, in order to minimise the opportunity for somebody to take a photo of her and perhaps place it on social media sites for other users to mock.

Amanda also talks about avoiding spaces, but this time where she is likely to encounter the younger generation who are likely to use dwarf representations as a form of insult:

> *I don't go to MacDonald's [fast food chain], I don't like the food, but not only that, you get a lot of young people there and they can be just awful. They all like to have a good giggle at you with their friends, and you will always get that one person trying to show off by calling you some name like midget or again asking where Snow White is (Amanda).*

The vast majority of participants mentioned receiving unwanted attention from teenagers, especially when the teenagers are in groups because the teenagers were more likely to cause unwanted attention. Of course, not all teenagers are going to provoke unwanted attention, but because of past experiences with teenagers, Amanda will try and minimise any risk of encountering any more unwanted attention, which Steve further talks about:

> *Have you experienced any times when these stereotypes have been directed at you? (Erin)*
> *I was going to a gym, it was in the leisure centre and was right next door to a comprehensive school and the time that my gym class was finishing was the school's lunchtime. I was coming out of the gym as they were coming*

*out of the school, and nothing directly at me but I could hear the circus
tune being whistled as I walked towards the car, and I just took no notice
of it and just carried on (Steve)*

Snow White sort of tune as well (Joan)

*I just didn't go back there. I don't need to put myself in that position
(Steve)*

It spoilt something for Steve (Joan)

*Yeah, and it was working as I was losing weight. But I stopped going and
found another gym (Steve)*

These timings (gym classes/school lunch break) are created by non-disabled
people, but due to how cultural representations influence unwanted encounters, Steve must find an alternative in order to pursue a leisure activity.
Although Steve has found another gym, demonstrating a good alternative, it
means he is restricted on which gym he can go to due to unwanted social
behaviour which is clearly influenced by humorous representations of
dwarfism. His level of choice is restricted, which places him in an unequal
position within society. Grace further points how representations, that have
constructed stereotypes of dwarfism, can restrict where she chooses to go:

*Have you experienced any times when these stereotypes have been used
towards you? (Erin)*

*Yeah, when people are drunk. I have learnt to ignore it. I still go into pubs
near where I live, but I wouldn't risk going to pubs in other areas. I am
always worried that it could start off with name-calling and then turn into
physical abuse (Grace)*

The majority of participants spoke about how they received more unwanted
attention from people who were under the influence of alcohol. When people
are drunk, they tend to act in ways that they would not if they were sober.
Shakespeare, (1999) suggests that jokes towards disabled people are more
likely to emerge when people are drunk, as drunkenness leads to social rules
being ignored. Drinking spaces, such as pubs and bars, encourage people to
get drunk and socialise due to the meaning of the space. The meaning of
these spaces also makes unwanted social behaviour more acceptable. This is
not to say that all behaviours will be tolerated, but that jokes towards people
with dwarfism, which are associated with representations, will be more
acceptable. We only have to remember that the 'sport' known as *'dwarf
tossing'* originated in a bar in Australia. Grace points out that the stereotypes associated with dwarfism have been used towards her, in the form
of name-calling, and this prevents her from going to new pubs. Cultural
stereotypes of dwarfism clearly stimulant to negative behaviour. Several
participants pointed out that they preferred to visit local or familiar places
as they were less likely to receive unwanted attention from people who knew
them or were used to their presence. Being familiar to other people helps to

challenge dominant stereotypes associated with dwarfism. It also allows people with dwarfism to be familiar with other people, whereas they cannot be sure how strangers will react to their presence.

Overall in this section, it is apparent that avoidance of spaces is affected by how other members of the public react towards people with dwarfism, often relating to cultural representations of dwarfism. This section has demonstrated that spaces are not always disabling because of the physicality of a space, but due to an attitudinal environment which disables people who look different (Hawkesworth, 2001). Goffman, (1963) suggests that the stigmatised can never be certain of how the 'normal' person may react to their presence, and therefore the stigmatised person may arrange their life in order to avoid such confrontation. The unwanted attention people with dwarfism receive within public spaces effects where they choose to access, as they often avoid places where they perceive they will receive unwanted attention. The strategy of avoidance aids in limiting how much psycho-emotional disablism they experience, but it also limits their equal standing in society as they cannot access the same spaces in the same way as non-disabled people.

Being aware of what social restraints may be encountered is affected by past experiences, which in turn lead to feelings of anxiety which influence people with dwarfism to avoid particular spaces. Knowing where to avoid is determined by who may be occupying that space, if they have received unwanted attention in that space before, or if it is likely to contain particular representations of dwarfism. Improving representations of dwarfism could help to change how people perceive and subsequently interact with people with dwarfism.

5.5 Challenging cultural representations and changing attitudes

As previously shown, cultural representations of dwarfism can encourage unwanted attention from other members of the public, including mockery, which can subsequently result in people with dwarfism avoiding particular areas of the built environment. Adelson, (2005a) argues that there is a decreasing acceptance of dwarfs being employed within certain entertainment industries, such as being hired out for stag dos, due to how they socially construct dwarfs. Although people with dwarfism are still employed in low bar entertainment, which is based on exploiting their height, Adelson, (2005a) documents how many people with dwarfism are now employed within regular jobs. Adelson, (2005a) focuses on the advocacy work being employed by people with dwarfism in the present day to try to give dwarfism a more positive identity. Pushing for more positive representations of dwarfism can aid in increasing their equality within society. With this important change within employment, it is also beneficial to focus on how people with dwarfism think cultural representations can be used to promote a more positive representation of dwarfism, which reflects the changing lives of people with dwarfism. Longmore (2003: 145) argues that positive media images of disability 'reflect the growing socio-political perception of disabled people as a minority group and the increasing impact of the disability civil rights movement'. However, as previously discussed, people with dwarfism are often on the margins of the disabled community.

One of the main ideas proposed to improve representations of dwarfism in media is to provide people with dwarfism with more serious or true-to-life roles to play, as opposed to being a figure of fun:

> ... *I think what we need to do is put out more positive images. I was quite proud of Eastenders [popular British soap opera] when they cast a dwarf as a teacher, and I loved that (Anne).*

> *It would be nice to see more dwarfs playing characters like the one in Eastenders instead of always being the fool. I think it would make some people realise that we are not all stupid and that we have normal lives. A lot of dwarfs have normal jobs, but that is not shown, and so people just think we are all panto actors (Amanda).*

> *There are some and I think that's good. There is a little person in Eastenders (Joan)*
> *Wasn't she a teacher? (Steve)*
> *Yes (Joan)*
> *We do need more in more serious roles, that would be a good thing (Steve)*
> *They have actors with Down's syndrome which is good, and people in chairs [wheelchairs], that's fine, and I think our community can do that (Joan)*
> *I think it would make the public see us in a different light, and they would take us more seriously (Steve)*

British soap operas, such as EastEnders, are based on people living in British society, and although they may not truly represent British life, due to their often over dramatised storylines, showing a character with dwarfism as a school teacher can be seen as a more varied portrayal of dwarfism, in comparison to something from mythology or someone to laugh at. Sancho, (2003) suggests that by showing disabled people on television with minimal focus on their disability, but shown in a way which portrays them as being just like anyone else in society, helps to increase acceptance towards them. Having a person with dwarfism playing the role of an everyday person helps to challenge misconceptions of dwarfism, especially when appearing in a popular soap opera seen by millions of people living in the UK. A character with dwarfism working as a school teacher subtly challenges the belief that entertainment work is the only occupation people with dwarfism can fulfil. Everyday roles would give less novelty value to their height and help to show other members of the public that stereotypes such as humour are not related to their height. 'Producing films with realistic portrayals of disabled people can help to change the attitudes of other members of the public towards disabled people' (Schwartz, et al., 2010: 842). This can encourage dwarfism to be read differently which may result in less unwanted attention for people with dwarfism in society.

Showing dwarfism in a more challenging way would offer the chance of normality. Other participants also spoke about the potential documentaries have in challenging stereotypes:

> *That is one of the reasons we made that documentary to try and get over the myths and to show people the reality (Jade).*

> *I think it is more to do with awareness. A lot of people need to watch the documentaries and not make the programme funny. I think it will give them a very different picture of us. I think TV programmes more than anything need to change as a lot or people watch TV (Myraar).*

Producing more documentaries on dwarfism can be seen as a productive way of challenging the representations that exist by having a more realistic re-presentation of dwarfism. Reality shows featuring people with dwarfism can help to 'destigmatise' them by showing them as ordinary people (Backstrom, 2012). This can include them being engaged in everyday activities, including raising a family and being in regular employment, as opposed to en-tertainment spectacles which fail to offer the chance of normality (Darke, 2004). In order to counteract the negative representation of people with dwarfism, including the ones that showed dwarfism as something different, the participants suggested showing more documentaries or placing actors with dwarfism in roles which did not focus or ridicule their height. Documentaries aim to distribute information about their subject, in this case dwarfism, in order to change the viewers' attitudes and opinions towards the subject (Garland-Thomson, 2002). This is especially beneficial when the subject is an uncommon sight within society.

Although documentaries can help to show the real lives of people with dwarfism, challenging dominant representations, Askcharity, (2006) sug-gests that particular documentaries, such as 'shock docs' can have a negative effect upon the people they are about. In their study, Askcharity, (2006) found that documentaries that focused on people with abnormal bodies, such as children with Progeria, a genetic condition that accelerates old age, had a more negative effect upon disabled people. This would relate to both Kayleigh and Amanda who spoke about one particular documentary about dwarfism which they thought had the unwanted result of perpetuating the stereotype of humour and amusement linked to dwarfism, as opposed to fighting it:

> *I couldn't watch that seven dwarfs programme. The trailer looked so silly, and again something just about our height and how you can laugh at it.*

It is meant to be a reality show, but again the dwarfs in it were just making fun of their height (Amanda).

I am very concerned about what Channel Four is bringing out, the reality TV show based on a Panto [Pantomime] … as it just feeds into the myth that everybody who has dwarfism works in Panto (Kayleigh).

The show Amanda and Kayleigh are referring to focuses on a group of performers with dwarfism getting ready for a pantomime, in which they play the seven dwarfs from *Snow White and the Seven Dwarfs*. This reinforces the stereotype that all people with dwarfism take part in the annual pantomimes. Both Amanda and Kayleigh think the show can have a negative effect upon people with dwarfism because it encourages the audience to laugh at the dwarfs. The show reinforces people's idea of people with dwarfism being an object of ridicule within society, instead of showing people with dwarfism in a more positive light and providing a more realistic portrayal. Although some people with dwarfism may take part in pantomimes, not all of them do. None of the participants interviewed mentioned taking part in a pantomime, including Kayleigh who works as an actress. Adelson, (2005b) explores how people with dwarfism are rejecting employment within lowbrow entertainment, including within pantomimes, resulting in companies having to cast dwarf actors from other European countries. People with dwarfism are now able to gain employment within a myriad of occupations due to better disability equality. Although reality shows may be a good way of challenging and changing people's attitudes towards people with dwarfism, the shows have to challenge the stereotypes instead of playing on them. A reality show, which gives a false representation of people with dwarfism, reinforces the idea that people with dwarfism are acceptable to ridicule. The name 'reality' implies that the shows are true to life, creating a false perception of their content. Backstrom, (2012) points out that reality shows can act as a replacement to the freak show. If reality shows are now acting as a replacement to the freak shows then they are still promoting people with dwarfism as spectacles. This is not to suggest that documentaries cannot help to change attitudes but rather that caution is needed in order to not present a documentary which resembles more of a modern-day freak show, rather than an educational programme which gives an everyday representation of dwarfism. Whilst Backstrom, (2012) argues that reality shows can help to 'destigmatise' dwarfism, it must be noted that it depends on the content of the reality show and how it represents people with dwarfism.

5.6 Conclusion

This chapter has explored the cultural representations of people with dwarfism, including within popular culture and mass media. Even with improved disability equality, people with dwarfism are still deemed inferior through how they are exploited within the entertainment industry. Representations of dwarfism are underpinned by ableism, which renders the small body inferior and thus acceptable to ridicule. Present-day representations do not seem to have changed much since the European courts or Victorian freak shows. It is not enough to get rid of the freaks shows, but rather the form of exploitation they encouraged needs to be eradicated. Cultural myths and images can influence how people view and come to understand disability. In the entertainment industry, people with dwarfism are constructed as humours and mythic, as opposed to disabled people. People with dwarfism have expressed that representations of people with dwarfism contribute to the social barriers that they encounter and thus can be seen as a contributing factor to their disablement within the built environment. This resonates with the agenda-setting theory, as audiences are influenced by representations of people with dwarfism. Having a more varied set of representations can help to challenge the stereotypical portrayal of people with dwarfism as oddities or figures of fun. The chapter has demonstrated the various ways that dominant representations of dwarfism can be challenged in order to give a more positive and varied portrayal of dwarfism which in turn can help to change how people interact with people with dwarfism. Even humorous representations can exist, providing they are disability humour as opposed to disabling humour. However, these representations need to outweigh the negative representations.

Whilst dwarfism continues to be exploited by the entertainment industry and constructed as inferior, people with dwarfism will continue to have unequal access to the built environment. The unwanted attention that people with dwarfism experience as a result of cultural representation affects how they negotiate public spaces, including avoiding spaces due to the representation of particular spaces. Social barriers experienced by people with dwarfism, as a result of cultural representations, result in experiences of psycho-emotional disablism. The disablist impact of cultural representations needs to be given as much attention as the physically disabling barriers that people with dwarfism encounter.

Notes

1 The film made an estimated $392 million at the box office.
2 *Austin Powers: The Spy who Shagged Me* grossed at the global box office (BoxOfficeMojo, 2020a).

6 Conclusion

The politics of space, identity and the sized body

6.1 Introduction

This book originates from the realisation that research concerning lives of people with dwarfism was limited. I have attempted to broaden the research on the lives of people with dwarfism and contribute to existing research, including Adelson, (2005a, 2005b), Kruse, (2002, 2003, 2010) and Shakespeare, et al. (2007, 2010). This book has explored the social and spatial experiences of people with dwarfism. Now what is required is determining how equal access can be obtained for people with dwarfism. This involves changing the representations of spaces, cultural representations of dwarfism and disability perceptions. This book provides a deeper understanding of how people with a particular impairment experience public spaces by exploring the socio-spatial experiences of people with dwarfism in order to expand knowledge on dwarfism and within several different academic subjects. An intersectional approach has been utilised by engaging with the subjects of Human Geography and Disability Studies to shows a number of empirical the disabling experiences people with dwarfism encounter in their daily lives. This book makes a number of empirical contributions which can be applied to Geographies of Disabilities, Social Geographies of Body Size, and Disability Studies.

As noted in the introduction, this book has revolved around dwarfism's most prominent features: body size and shape. It has not focused on secondary impairments, however, they have been discussed where relevant. Giving less attention to more well recognised functional limitations, such as mobility impairments, has allowed this book to demonstrate how non-normative body sizes are disabled within society. This book has exposed the numerous disabling barriers people with dwarfism experience, demonstrating that 'just being small' has big implications for people with dwarfism.

This concluding chapter is separated into several sections that summarise the main findings. The first part of the chapter summarises the importance of engaging with spatial theories in order to understand how people with dwarfism navigate through different spaces and the different strategies they employ when negotiating different spaces, including avoidance and doing things differently. As a result, this section proposes how Universal Design is beneficial for people with dwarfism and why it needs more consideration when designing spaces. The next section focuses on disability identity and dwarfism, which aids in understanding the importance of adopting a social model based identity of disability. Moving on, as this book has focused on body size, it is important to understand how this work contributes to geographies of body size. The last part of the chapter offers ways to challenge current cultural representations of dwarfism. As not all experiences of people with dwarfism can be explored in one book, the possible future research directions that stem from this book are lastly discussed.

6.2 Dwarfism and the politics of space

The notion of space is important in understanding how people with dwarfism navigate through the built environment and interact with different spaces. Drawing on the work of Imrie, (1996b, 1997, 1999), this book has shown, with particular reference to chapter 1, how spaces created for the average-sized, able-bodied person are disabling for people with dwarfism. Using Lefebvre's triad of space, this book has shown how the spatial practices that people with dwarfism adopt are influenced by the representational space and the representations of space (meaning and materiality). The representations of space construct the socio-spatial barriers that people with dwarfism encounter.

The social-spatial barriers relate to specific norms in the human population. Constructing spaces to accommodate for the majority is a cost-effective way of conceiving spaces, however, it excludes the minority from society. As a result, there are now minimal accommodations for people with dwarfism in the form of accessible spaces. The socio-spatial barriers that people with dwarfism encounter are more complex than just socio-spatial barriers that are the result of public spaces being created for the average-sized, able-bodied person. The barriers also show that spaces created for other groups within society, including children and other impairments, can also be a contributing factor to their disablement. This demonstrates that the representation of a space influences its production, which subsequently influences the spatial practices of people with dwarfism.

The representation of an accessible space is influenced by society's perception of disability. Disability is often conceived as a functional limitation, or more specifically, a mobility impairment which requires the use of a mobility aid. This impacts the meaning of a space (representational) and consequently the spatial practice of people with dwarfism. Whilst accessible spaces are mostly suitable for people with dwarfism, whom they are constructed for can be disabling in the same way as creating public spaces for the average-sized, able-bodied person. There is a normalcy of disability which results in creating accessible spaces for specific disabled people. This is reflective of a neoliberal agenda, which aims to reduce costs. This contributes to Imrie, (1996b, 1997) who criticises the implementation of disabled spaces for wheelchair users whilst ignoring the needs of other impairments. When implementing spaces for different users, it is important to take into account what impact they may have on other users.

As shown, spaces adapted for children often create socio-spatial barriers for people with dwarfism. This is particularly problematic in spaces specifically for children, such as playgrounds, as many people with dwarfism have their own children, some of whom also have dwarfism, and thus it is important to recognise how people with dwarfism deal with socio-spatial barriers that are associated with parenting. This would include exploring how child facilities impact how parents with dwarfism care for their children. How do they cope with using a pram and public changing facilities for infants? As well as socio-spatial barriers, it would also be interesting to focus on the attitudes they have encountered as parents, such as are they deemed suitable parents due to their dwarfism? Some of these issues were touched upon in a few interviews but were not explored deep enough to incorporate within this book.

6.2.1 The significance of avoidance

As pointed out, within Geographies of Disabilities, disability is not only about physically inaccessible spaces but also about an attitudinal environment which can affect access to particular spaces (Butler and Bowlby, 1997; Laws, 1994; Hawksworth, 2001). As Hawksworth, (2001) shows in her research, bodily differences can lead to social disablement, including unwanted attitudes and the avoidance of particular spaces. Due to their bodily difference, people with dwarfism encounter social attitudes which can lead to the avoidance of various spaces. This avoidance impacts on their equality within society.

- Do people with dwarfism avoid certain spaces in order to avoid negative social situations?

People with dwarfism often choose to avoid certain spaces due to socio-spatial barriers and social barriers. Avoidance is the result of ableism within society. Ableism takes many forms and has numerous implications for people with dwarfism in society, which for a long time have been ignored. The social barriers people with dwarfism encounter are the result of disablist attitudes which result in psycho-emotional disablism. Avoiding spaces reduces psycho-emotional disablism, but as a consequence, people with dwarfism are restricted in their full participation within society.

Through engaging with how cultural representations affect people with dwarfism, this book has shown that people with dwarfism actively avoid spaces where they perceive they will encounter negative social situations. There are specific spaces which are often associated with cultural representations of dwarfism, such as the cinema showing a film featuring a character with dwarfism, which some people with dwarfism avoid.

6.2.2 *Other forms of resistance*

Avoidance of particular spaces, dependency, doing something differently and socially interacting with other members of the public in ways to counteract disabling attitudes are all forms of agency which allow people with dwarfism to minimise the number of socio-spatial barriers and social barriers they encounter. These situations were space/time dependent, as people with dwarfism are often reluctant to overcome a socio-spatial barrier in certain space or at a certain time, for example when a space is busier.

People with dwarfism employ their own agency to deal with disabling barriers, revealing a more complex view into their experiences. The agency involved includes both overcoming a socio-spatial barrier in their own way and dealing with social barriers which often result in subtle forms of disablism. Subtle forms of disablism relate to how other members of the public respond to people with dwarfism, which may not purposely be offensive, such as making an unwanted remark when doing something differently, however they demonstrate an unequal power relation.

• Due to unaccommodating infrastructure how do people with dwarfism negotiate socio-spatial barriers?

People with dwarfism use a number of ways to respond to socio-spatial barriers, such as through avoidance, dependency or doing something differently. This book has shown that spaces which are not size-suitable can leave people with dwarfism more dependent on other members of the public. Being more dependent on others is not straightforward but involves various social responses, including from helpfulness to being ignored. To give a more complex understanding of how dependency relations are played out within public spaces, this book explored the notion of interdependence. This involved not only understanding their degree of dependency but how other members of the public socially interact with people with dwarfism when they require assistance. Asking for assistance is not a straightforward interaction but is affected by how other members of the public react to these situations. This work contributes to how disabled people manage social interactions and illustrates some of the ways in which other members of the public respond to the presence of disabled people in public spaces. Dependency for people with dwarfism is due to the inaccessibility of public spaces, and independence can only come about if the correct assistance is given or if they are provided with more height suitable facilities. Interdependency is about ensuring that the correct assistance is provided, such as not receiving unwanted remarks or being ignored and ensuring a person's choice is not impinged when requiring assistance.

Dependency and doing something differently are dependent upon the socio-spatial barrier, including whether or not a person with dwarfism can overcome it in their own way. For example, some have their own way of getting on a bar stool, but they do not have any way to be able to reach an item off a high shelf and thus have to ask someone for assistance. This leads to the second research question:

• What social responses do people with dwarfism experience when dealing with socio-spatial barriers within public spaces?

This book has shown that when people with dwarfism use their own way of overcoming a socio-spatial barrier that it can invite unwanted attention, relating to work of Keith, (1996) and Scully, (2010). People with dwarfism employ a number of ways to not only deal with socio-spatial barriers but also when socially interacting with other members of the public in order to receive assistance or to minimise the unwanted attention they get when performing a task differently. This further adds to Hansen and Philo, (2007) by showing how responding to different socio-spatial barriers, in their own way, can provoke unwanted attention as they do not match ableist expectations. In order for people with dwarfism to be able to fully overcome socio-spatial barriers, it is not always about changing the space to accommodate them, but ensuring that other members of the public have the right attitude towards them doing something differently or when asking for help. If not, then people with dwarfism are likely to avoid interacting with an inaccessible space, which impinges upon their equal access to the built environment.

6.2.3 *Universal design and inclusive spaces*

It is important to consider how spaces can be made more accommodating for people with dwarfism. The built environment can become more accessible for people with dwarfism through the implementation of different design practices including Universal Design. Universal Design is based upon the principle that there is only one population, comprised of individuals representing diverse characteristics and abilities (Iwarsson and Stahl, 2003). It would aid in changing the representation of a space, as Universal Design takes place from the design and planning stage of a new space.

Universal Design is defined as 'the design of products and environments to be usable by all people, to the greatest extent possible, without the need for adaptation or specialized design' (Mace, 1985 in Steinfeld and Masel, 2012). Universal Design is based upon the principle that there is only one population, comprised of individuals representing diverse characteristics and abilities (Iwarsson and Stahl, 2003). Universal Design is about accommodating for everyone and thus spaces would be suitable for a diverse range of bodies. This would mean less of a need for separate accessible spaces. As shown, accessible spaces are not always accessible for people with dwarfism due to them being created for a narrow range of impairments. If more spaces are generally accessible for a wider range of people, there is less of a need for accessible spaces, removing the social and spatial barriers people with dwarfism encounter when accessing them.

Universal Design consists of seven design principles (ibid). Principle seven of Universal Design focuses on the needs of different body sizes:

> *Design Principle Seven—Size and Space: for Approach and Use. Appropriate size and space is designed for approach, reach, manipulation, and use, regardless of the users body size, posture or mobility (Centre for Universal Design 1997 in Steinfeld and Maisel, 2012: 12).*

Universal Design would provide a way to show how spaces can be made to accommodate for people with dwarfism, such as through the implementation of multi-level or adjustable facilities which benefit a range of body sizes. This book has shown what spaces are disabling for people with dwarfism, whereas Universal Design can be used to show how they can be made enabling. Whilst principle 7 of Universal Design does promise hope, it needs to be ensured that this access again does not solely favour wheelchair users. Of course, the needs of wheelchair users should be included, however, provisions such as reach will not benefit people with dwarfism if measurements are based on a typical wheelchair user. The ergonomics of a space would need to be based on the average statue of a person with dwarfism, as opposed to the average wheelchair user who is taller. However, it would still need to take into account the ergonomics of a taller person in order to provide equal access for all.

6.3 Dwarfism, the social model of disability and disability identity

Whilst it is often argued that dwarfism is more of a difference than a disability, this argument becomes obsolete when adopting the social model of disability. Dwarfism is an impairment that does result in a different body size, however, this difference is disabled in a one-size-fits-all society. This aids in broadening our understanding of disability by including the experiences of body size as an impairment.

* Do accessible spaces help or hinder people with dwarfism in their negotiation of socio-spatial barriers?

As demonstrated in chapter 1, accessible spaces both help and hinder people with dwarfism in their negotiations of socio-spatial barriers. The accessibility of these spaces is affected by for whom they are constructed, which relates to perceptions of disability. Whilst accessible spaces can aid people with dwarfism in their negotiation of socio-spatial barriers, most people with dwarfism thought that the reason for this was because of the coincidence in meeting a wheelchair user's needs which is often a case of facilities needing to be lower. It is these lower facilities, such as low counters, which help people with dwarfism in their negotiation of socio-spatial barriers, including high counters. Accessible spaces, in some cases, can impede access, particularly when sinks have been implemented for wheelchair users, which may be low but are wider in order for the wheelchair to fit underneath. This means that because of their shorter arm length, people with dwarfism cannot reach the taps and thus still encounter a disabling situation. Thus the implementation of accessible spaces does not mean increased access for people with dwarfism, but can present another disabling space.

Currently, there are limited access provisions made for people with dwarfism. Accommodating for wheelchair users does not provide equal access for people with dwarfism. Building legislation pertaining to disability, such as Part M of the Buildings and Regulations Act (2010), needs to broaden and include the access needs of people with dwarfism. This requires dwarfism to be more readily recognised as a disability.

Accessing accessible spaces is often met with difficulties as people with dwarfism are not always seen as the correct users of these spaces. This corresponds to Shakespeare, et al. (2010) who point out that the cultural representations of dwarfism fail to show it as an actual disability. The debate as to who is, or is not disabled, has often been constructed using crude policy and representational (media) binaries (Briant, et al., 2011), ones that assume disability is fixed, static, knowable and easily measured.

It must be acknowledged that whilst the social model has aided in changing how disability is conceptualised, this has not been universal. The social model of disability does not seem to be as well-known within society as it is within academia. Furthermore, general society is reliant on being able to identify disabled people through obvious indicators, such as a mobility aid. This has implications for people with dwarfism, including how they are treated. It is interesting that when people with dwarfism use a wheelchair or mobility scooter that they receive less unwanted attention, suggesting a hierarchy of impairments. This hierarchy manifests in different ways, including access to accessible spaces, resources and possibly disability benefits.

Dwarfism needs to be more widely recognised as a disability. A clearer disability status, such as the inclusion of dwarfism in disability images and within disability legislation, would aid in providing better access to equality. This would require people with dwarfism to positively adopt a disability identity. There are numerous factors as to why people with dwarfism do not identify themselves as a disabled people. Internalised ableism is the main factor in people with dwarfism not recognising themselves as disabled. They are forced to accept society's perception of them as 'just little'. Being challenged when trying to access accessible spaces is a subtle message that over time tells them that they are not disabled. Other media messages that construct disability as pitiful and tragic also impinge upon their identity as a disabled person. Due to disability often being associated with loss and being constructed as lesser, many people with dwarfism choose not to recognise themselves as disabled people. People with dwarfism should be recognised as a group of disabled people. This does not mean placing a stigmatising label upon them, but rather recognising that disability is a product of society.

This can aid in receiving appropriate support, such as better access and access to benefits which cover the extra costs associated with being disabled.

With the introduction of the Conservative–Liberal Democrat Coalition agreement in 2010, the UK has undergone major welfare reforms. These welfare reforms are having a significant impact upon disabled people (Stewart, 2016). Genuine disabled people are being denied a disability status, which would otherwise provide them with access to disability benefits. As Shakespeare, et al. (2010) assert, people with dwarfism are less likely to receive disability benefits than other disabled people, and yet they suggest that people with dwarfism could benefit from the support. Disabled people in the UK who receive the higher rate of the mobility component of Disability Living Allowance (DLA) can use the support to purchase a car, with the possibility of receiving support with the needed adjustments to be able to drive, e.g. pedal extensions. As this research has shown and as Kruse, (2003) points out, cars are a more suitable form of transportation for people with dwarfism because cars minimise the amount of unwanted social attention people with dwarfism receive, as well as removing the socio-spatial difficulties they encounter on public transport. Demos, (2004) suggests that, even if public transport was fully accessible, disabled people are often fearful of using it due to social attitudes. As this book has shown, people with dwarfism encounter a lot of unwanted attention, and thus a car can provide a more suitable alternative for commuting.

DLA has now been replaced with a new form of support called Personal Independent Payments (PIPs). All disabled people are being reassessed, in-cluding those on DLA indefinitely. Those on DLA indefinitely have long-term impairments, such as dwarfism and have been medically assessed and diagnosed, and thus reassessments have been criticized as uneconomical and timewasting. As figures show, only 0.5% of DLA claims are fraudulent (Stewart, 2016) and thus have been again criticized as uneconomical and an attack on disabled people. One requirement for PIPs is to be unable to walk more than 20 m, regardless of the person's difficulties walking. Again, a presumption is that to be disabled is to have a severe mobility impairment and thus most likely to be using a wheelchair. This does not mean that people with dwarfism can carry their shopping more than 20 m, run for a bus or not struggle to get onto a train. However, those who do not meet their stereotypical perception of disability are not going to receive the economic assistance they may need to get a car. In fact, Shakespeare, et al. (2010) suggest that having a car and being able to park closer to a supermarket removes the disabling task of having to carry heavy shopping bags. It also means that people with dwarfism do not have to push large trolleys across a busy car park. Despite this, even disabled parking bays are more likely to be more than 20 m away from the supermarket entrance, demonstrating that the 20 m requirement does not match the actual distances disabled people have to make. This new corporeal economy, one arguably driven by the retraction of the welfare state, has led to a number of major jeopardies, especially for those people who do not fit stereotyped images of disability (Boyd, 2012). Further research could focus on the impact current benefit changes are having on people with dwarfism.

6.4 Dwarfism and geographies of body size

This book aids in expanding knowledge within the subject of Geographies of Body Size by demonstrating how the small body interacts with different spaces, contributing to Hopkins, (2012) call for the discipline to expand and include other body sizes. Academic research, within Geographies of Body Size, which argues for fatness to be recognised as an impairment due to the way public spaces are unaccommodating for their body size, can be expanded to include dwarfism. Cooper, (1997) and Aphramor, (2009) consider fatness not to be recognised as a disability as it is seen as blameworthy. Whilst this may be true, not recognising body size as a disability is more complex and involves other factors, including stereotypical images of disability, which often includes a mobility aid. A dwarf's body size and shape should be recognised as an impairment due to the socio-spatial barriers they encounter, as well as the social responses towards their bodily appearance which often affect their negotiation of public spaces.

Using the social model of disability, this book contributes and expands on how having a body size which does not meet normal standards of size is disabled within public spaces (Aphramor, 2009; Chan and Gillick, 2005; Cooper, 1997; Longhurst, 2010). It relates to the ergonomics of a space and the facilities within it. This includes counters which are too high and facilities which are inaccessible because they accommodate for a particular standard of size. Different body sizes, which exceed the norm in different ways, are disabled in a one-size-fits-all society.

6.5 Challenging cultural representations of dwarfism

Blatant forms of disablism can include name-calling, which often relates to cultural representations of dwarfism. As shown in chapter 4, people with dwarfism are constructed as spectacles or mythical beings, which ignores the disabling aspects of dwarfism. These representations are a form of disablism, however, they go unchallenged. A more prominent disability identity would help to challenge some of the derogatory representations of dwarfism. Other disabled people are not represented in the same way as people with dwarfism. Certain forms of entertainment, such as dwarf tossing, are unique to them. A disability identity may make some forms of derogatory entertainment more ethically questionable. Would entertainment industries be as keen to promote dwarf entertainment if dwarf tossing was also known as disabled person tossing? Would somebody be as keen to hire out a disabled person for their stag do? Taking into account how cultural representations of dwarfism, especially those which humiliate people with dwarfism, impact upon the dignity of people with dwarfism in society aids in questioning the ethical implications of these representations. Challenging these representations would aid in changing how people with dwarfism are perceived and subsequently treated within society.

- Do cultural representations of dwarfism affect society's treatment towards people with dwarfism?

Using the agenda-setting theory, it can be suggested that constant images within the media, which in this case is dwarfism as something to laugh at or being portrayed as not quite human, influence other members of the public to perceive people with dwarfism in the same way. This book has shown that people with dwarfism think more varied representations of dwarfism would help to change how other members of the public perceive them, resulting in more positive interactions. This book gives a broader understanding of how cultural representations of dwarfism impact the spatial navigation of people with dwarfism. Exploring these representations has aided in providing another dimension as to how and why people with dwarfism experience public spaces differently from other members of the public.

There is also plenty of scope for questioning why some people with dwarfism still take part in entertainment which exploits their size and thus gains the other side of the story. Backstrom, (2012) points out that people with dwarfism who partake in shows which exploit their height claim that they are reaping the benefits, which can be assumed are economical, of professional display. However, solely partaking in derogatory entertainment for economic benefits does not take into account possible other factors. Interviewing dwarf entertainers and understanding their reasons, including understanding their socio-economic background, educational background and their general reasons for wanting to pursue a career which others deem exploitive would aid in providing a broader view of why dwarf entertainment still persists.

It is important that the ethical implications of dwarf entertainment take into consideration the psycho-emotional impact upon people with dwarfism in society. Whilst most people defend the career choices of some people with dwarfism, they overlook the wider implications for people with dwarfism in society. Van Etten, (1988) hypothetically argues that if five people partake in lowbrow entertainment (such as dwarf tossing), but ten people with dwarfism encounter the unwanted social repercussions as a result, then the entertainment becomes unacceptable. It is appropriate to assume that there are more people being negatively impacted by derogatory representations of dwarfism than there are benefiting from it.

6.6 New research directions

When people with dwarfism were being interviewed, several spoke about serious incidents that could be classed as a disability hate crime. As I did not specifically ask people with dwarfism about these kinds of incidents, there may be more to uncover. These incidents were a lot worse than the social barriers they spoke about, such as name-calling, because the persons were threatening. In one case, an average-sized man demanded money from a woman with dwarfism because the perpetrator was able to overpower her. Due to their body size, it can be questioned whether people with dwarfism are targeted due to their perceived vulnerability. In the UK, there is growing concern about disabled people being the targets of hate crimes, with a particular focus on people with learning difficulties due to the high rates of targeted abuse towards them. Focusing on dwarfism can help to expand research concerning disability hate crimes and further unpack why disabled people are targeted.

When speaking to the people with dwarfism, most were in employment, yet some spoke about how other people, including family members and social services, felt that when they were growing up they would not be employable or that they would only be suitable for particular kinds of employment. Obviously there will be various forms of employment that people with dwarfism will not be able to pursue due to their impairment, but further research could be carried out to explore any discriminatory attitudes towards them when seeking employment or within the workplace, including those possibly influenced by cultural representations of dwarfism. Kruse, (2002) shows in his paper that people with dwarfism are discriminated against when seeking employment due to their dwarfism. This would be interesting to look into further and to explore how people with dwarfism negotiate the labour market and the attitudes they have experienced when it comes to finding employment.

Various researchers have explored employment opportunities and discrimination in relation to disability and point out that disabled people are often discriminated from various jobs and experience discrimination within the workplace (Barnes and Mercer, 2010; Duckett, 2000). In their research, Shakespeare, et al. (2007) suggest that social barriers affect the work potential of people with dwarfism. Some people with dwarfism pointed out that within the workplace they experienced social barriers, including practical jokes being played on their height. Although they may be employed, further research could explore how they manage in the workplace in regards to both socio-spatial barriers and social barriers.

Whilst the media, from Disney to the pantomime, construct people with dwarfism as happy people who are acceptable to treat as less than human, the real experiences of people with dwarfism, including their mental health, go unnoticed. Whilst it has not been explored in this book, the mental health of people with dwarfism needs more consideration. Since writing this book and being part of numerous groups for people with dwarfism on Facebook, I have become more aware of many people with dwarfism committing suicide. Whilst this could be for a myriad of reasons, the experiences related to dwarfism can also be a contributing factor. For a minority group, it seems that there are high incidences of suicide, which needs consideration. Constant messages that tell you that you do not belong, whether these are physical, such as inaccessible buildings, or representations in the media, such as spreading the message that people with dwarfism are less than human, have implications for people with dwarfism in society, including a negative impact on a person's mental health. Over time, without the right support, these implications can grow and become a lot more problematic.

References

Abberley, P. (1997) The concept of oppression and the development of a social theory of disability, In Barton, L. and Oliver, M. (Eds) *Disability Studies: Past, Present and Future.* Leeds: The Disability Press, pp. 160–178.

Ablon, J. (1990) Ambiguity and difference: families with dwarf children. *Social Science and Medicine, 30* (8), 879–887.

Adelson, B. M. (2005a) *The Lives of Dwarfs: Their Journey from Public Curiosity to Social Liberation.* New Jersey: Rutgers University Press.

Adelson, B. M. (2005b) The changing lives of archetypal 'Curiosities' – and echoes of the past. *Disability Studies Quarterly, 25* (3), 1–13.

Andrews, K. C. (2019) *The Overworked Consumer: Self-Checkouts, Supermarkets and the Do-it-Yourself Economy.* London: Lexington Press.

Aphramor, L. (2009) Disability and the anti-obesity offensive. *Disability and Society, 24* (7), 897–909.

Askcharity (2006) 'Modern day freak shows?' Available online: http://www.google.co.uk/url?sa=t&rct=j&q=&esrc=s&frm=1&source=web&cd=2&ved=0CCwQFjAB&url=http%3A%2F%2Fvamu.org.uk%2Fdownloads%2Fmodern_day_freak_shows.pdf&ei=696OUMOOBITK0QXpy4CgDg&usg=AFQjCNEXe_arWz3numOH8r11C0MwFVpZgw&sig2=6npG2HuHIJV88SlZvqlMfg (Accessed 04/10/2012).

Attride-Stirling, J. (2001) Thematic networks: an analytical tool for qualitative research. *Qualitative Research, 1* (3), 385–405.

Backstrom, L. (2012) From freak show to the living room: cultural representations of dwarfism and obesity. *Sociological Forum, 27* (3), 682–707.

Baker, K. and Donelly, M. (2001) The social experiences of children with disability and the influence of environment: a framework for intervention. *Disability and Society, 16* (1), 71–85.

Banks, M. (2007) *Using Visual Data in Qualitative Research.* London: Sage.

Barnes, C. (1991a) *Disabled People in Britain and Discrimination: A Case for Anti-Discrimination Legislation.* London: Hurst and Co Ltd.

Barnes, C. (1991b) *Disabling comedy and anti-discrimination legislation. Coalition,* (December) 26–28.

Barnes, C. (1992) *Disabling Imagery and the Media.* Krumlin: Ryburn Publishing.

Barnes, C. (1996) *The social model of disability: myths and misconceptions. Coalition,* (August) 27–33.

Barnes, C. (2011) Understanding disability and the importance of design for all. *Journal of Accessibility and Design for All, 1* (1), 55–80.

Barnes, C. (2012) Understanding the social model of disability, In Watson, N., Roulstone, A. and Thomas, C. (Eds) *Routledge Handbook of Disability Studies*. London: Routledge pp. 12–29.

Barnes, C. and Mercer, G. (2010) *Exploring Disability*. Cambridge: Polity Press.

Barnes, J. (1979) *Who Should Know What?* Harmondsworth: Penguin.

Basit, T. (2003) Manual or electronic? The role of coding in qualitative data analysis. *Educational Research, 45* (2),143–154.

Blaska, J. K. (2004) Children's literature that includes characters with disabilities or illness. *Disability Studies Quarterly, 24* (1). https://dsq-sds.org/article/view/854/1029.

Berger, R. (2013) Now I see it, now I don't: researcher's position and reflexivity in qualitative research. *Qualitative Research, 15*, 1–16.

Bickenbach, J., Chatterji, S., Badley, E. and Ustun, T. (1999) Models of disablement, universalism and the international classification of impairments, disabilities and handicaps. *Social Science and Medicine, 48* (9), 1173–1187.

Billig, M. (2005) *Laughter and ridicule: towards a social critique of humour*. London: Sage.

Bird, C. M. (2005) How I stopped dreading and learned to love transcription. *Qualitative Inquiry, 11* (2), 226–248.

Bogdon, R. (1988) *Freak Show*. Chicago: University of Chicago Press.

Bogdan, R. (1996) The social construction of freaks, In Garland-Thomson, R. (Eds) *Freakery: Cultural Spectacles of the Extraordinary Body*. London: New York University Press, pp. 23–37.

Bolt, D. (2014) *The Metanarrative of Blindness: A Re-Reading of Twentieth-Century Anglophone Writing*. University of Michigan Press: Ann Arbor.

Bolt, D. (2019) *Cultural Disability Studies in Education*. London: Routledge.

BoxOfficeMojo (2020a) Powers: The Spy who Shagged Me, *ImdbPro [online]* Available online: https://www.boxofficemojo.com/title/tt0145660/?ref_=bo_se_r_1 (Accessed 05/05/2020).

BoxOfficeMojo (2020b) Austin Powers in Goldmember, *ImdbPro [online]* Available online: https://www.boxofficemojo.com/release/rl944080385/?ref_=bo_frs_table_76 (Accessed 05/05/2020).

Boyd, V. (2012) "Are some disabilities more equal than others?" Conceptualising fluctuating or reoccuring impairments within contemporary legislation and practice. *Disability and Society, 27* (4), 459–469.

Braye, S., Dixon, K. and Gibbons. T. (2013) 'A mockery of equality': an exploratory investigation into disabled activists' views of the Paralympic games. *Disability and Society, 28* (7), 984–996.

Brandon, T. and Pritchard, G. (2011) "Being fat": a conceptual analysis using three models of disability. *Disability and Society, 26* (1), 79–92.

Briant, E., Watson, N. and Philo, G. (2011) *Bad News for Disabled People: How the Newspapers are Reporting Disability*. Glasgow, UK: Project Report. Strathclyde Centre for Disability Research and Glasgow Media Unit, University of Glasgow.

Butler, R. (1994) Geography and visually-impaired and blind populations. *Transactions of the Institute of British Geographers, 19* (3), 366–368.

Butler, R. and Bowlby, S. (1997) Bodies and spaces: an exploration of disabled people's experience of public space. *Environment and Planning D: Society and Space, 15* (4), 411–433.

Butler, R. and Parr, H. (1999) *Mind and Body Spaces*. London: Routledge.

Campbell, K. F. (2008) Exploring internalised ableism using critical race theory. *Disability and Society, 23* (2), 151–162.

Campbell, K. F. (2009) *Contours of Ableism: The Production of Disability and Abledness.* Basingstoke: Palgrave Macmillan.

Carmeli, Y. S. (1988) Wee Pea: the total play of the dwarf in the circus, *The Drama Review 3* (4), 128–145.

Chan, K. C. N. and Gillick, C. A. (2009) Fatness as a disability: questions of personal and group identity. *Disability and Society, 24* (2), 231–243.

Chouinard, V. (1999a) Life at the margins: Disabled women's explorations of ableist Spaces, In Kenworthy-Teather, E. (Eds) *Embodied Geographies: Spaces, Bodies and the Rights of Passage.* London: Routledge, pp. 142–156.

Chouinard, V. (1999b) Making space for disabling differences: challenging ableist geographies. *Environment and Planning D: Society and Space, 15* (1), 379–390.

Chouinard, V. (2000) Getting ethical: for inclusive and engaged geographies of disability. *Ethics, Place and Environment, 3* (1), 70–80.

Chouinard, V. and Grant, A. (1995) On being not even anywhere near 'the project': ways of putting ourselves in the picture. *Antipode, 27* (2), 137–166.

Chouinard, V., Hall, E. and Wilton, R. (2010) *Towards Enabling Geographies.* England: Ashgate.

Clark-Ibanez, M. (2004) Framing the social world with photo-elicitation exercises. *Qualitative research, 47* (12), 1507–1527.

Colls, R. (2004) 'Looking alright, feeling alright': emotions, sizing and the geographies of women's experiences of clothing consumption. *Social & Cultural Geography, 5* (4), 583–596.

Colls, R. (2006) Outsize/outside: bodily bigness and the emotional experiences of British women shopping for clothes. *Gender, Place and Culture, 13* (5), 529–545.

Cook, C. (2012) Email interviewing: generating data with a vulnerable population. *Journal of Advanced Nursing, 68* (6), 1330–1339.

Cooper, C. (1997) Can a fat woman call herself disabled? *Disability and Society, 12* (1), 31–41.

Crooks, I. and Chouinard, V. (2006) An embodied geography of disablement: chronically ill women's struggles for enabling places in spaces of health care and daily life. *Health and Place, 12* (3), 345–352.

Crook, I., Chouinard, V. and Wilton, R. (2008) Confronting, embracing, rejecting: women's negotiations of disability after the onset of chronic illness. *Social Science and Medicine, 67* (11), 1837–1846.

Crow, L. (1992) *Renewing the social model of disability. Coalition* (July) 5–9.

Crow, L. (1996) Including all of our lives: Renewing the social model of disability. In Morris, J. (Eds) *Encounters With Strangers.* London: The Women's Press, pp. 206–226.

Darke, P. (1994) The elephant man (David Lynch EMI Films, 1980): an analysis from a disabled perspective. *Disability and Society, 9* (3), 327–342.

Darke, A. P. (1998) Understanding cinematic representations of disability, In Shakespeare, T.(Eds) *The Disability Reader.* London: Continuum, pp. 181–198.

Darke, A. P. (2004) The changing face of representations of disability in the media, In Swain, J., French, S., Barnes, C. and Thomas, C. (Eds) *Disabling Barriers-Enabling Spaces* (second edition). London: Sage, pp. 100–105.

Davis, F. (1961) Deviance Disavowal: the management of strained interaction by the way the visibly handicapped. *Social Problems, 9* (2), 120–132.

Davis, L. J. (1995) *Enforcing Normalcy: Disability, Deafness and the Body*. London: Verso.

Davis, L. J. (2006) *The Disability Studies Reader*. Routledge: London.

Deal, M. (2003) Disabled people's attitudes towards other impairment groups: a hierarchy of impairments. *Disability and Society, 18* (7), 897–910.

Dear, M., Wilton, R., Gaber, L. G. and Takahashi, L. (1997) Seeing people differently: the socio-spatial construction of disability. *Environment and Planning D: Space and Society, 15* (4), 455–480.

Demos (2004) *Stories of Disablism*. London: Hendy Banks.

Derkensen, M. (2020) Induction and reception of dignity in Diego Velaquez's portraits of court dwarfs. *Journal of Literary and Cultural Disability Studies, 14* (2), 187–201.

Directgov (2012) Disability and the Equality Act 2010. Available online: http://www.direct.gov.uk/en/disabledpeople/rightsandobligations/disabilityrights/dg_4001068 (Accessed 31/05/2012).

Disability Discrimination Act (1995) (c.50), London, Available online: http://www.legislation.gov.uk/ukpga/1995/50/contents (Accessed 29/08/2013).

Dorn, M. and Laws, G. (1994) Social theory, body politics, and medical Geography: Extending Kearns's invitation. *The Professional Geographer, 46* (1), 106–110.

Doucet, A. and Mauther, N. S. (2006) Feminist methodologies and epistemologies In Clifton, D. Bryant, D. and Peck, L. (Eds) *Handbook of 21st Century Sociology*. Thousand Oaks, CA: Sage.

Driedger, M. S., Crooks, V. A. and Bennett, D. (2004) Engaging in the disablement process over space and Time: narratives of persons with Multiple Sclerosisin Ottawa, Canada. *The Canadian Geographer, 48* (2), 119–136.

Duckett, S. P. (2000) Disabled employment interviews: Warfare to work. *Disability and Society, 15* (7), 1019–1039.

Dyck, I. (1995) Hidden geographies: the changing lifeworlds of women with Multiple Sclerosis. *Social Science and Medicine, 40* (3), 307–320.

Dyck, I. (1999) Body troubles: women, the workplace and negotiations of a disabled identity, In Butler, R. and Parr, H. (Eds) *Mind and Body Spaces*. Abingdon: Routledge, pp. 119–137.

Dyck, I. (2000) Putting ethical research into practice: issues of context. *Ethics, Place and Environment, 3* (1), 80–87.

Edwards, C. (2013) Spacing access to justice: geographical perspectives on disabled people's interactions with the criminal justice system as victims of crime. *Area, 45* (3), 307–313.

Elwood, A. S. and Martin, D. G. (2000) "Placing" interviews: locations and scales of power in qualitative research. *Professional Geographer, 52* (4), 649–657.

England, K. V. L. (1994) Getting personal: reflexivity, positionality and feminist research. *The Professional Geographer, 46* (1) 80–89.

Esim, S. (1997) Can feminist methodology reduce power hierarchies in research settings? *Feminist Economics, 3* (2), 137–149.

Evans, B., Crooks, L. and Coaffee, J. (2012) Obesity, fatness and the city: critical urban geographies. *Geography Compass, 6* (2), 100–110.

Fereday, J. and Muir-Cochrane, E. (2006) Demonstrating rigour using thematic analysis: A hybrid approach of inductive and deductive coding and theme development, *International Journal of Qualitative Methods, 5* (1), 1–11.

Finkelstein, V. (1975) To deny or not to deny disability- What is disability? Available online: http://www.independentliving.org/docs1/finkelstein.html (Accessed 07/12/2012).

Finkelstein, V. (1980) *Attitudes and disabled people*. Available online: http://www.leeds.ac.uk/disability-studies/archiveuk/finkelstein/attitudes.pdf (Accessed: 10/02/2013).

Finkelstein, V. (1994) Getting there: non-disabling transport. Available online: http://disability-studies.leeds.ac.uk/files/library/finkelstein-Transport-Getting-There.pdf (Accessed 10/02/2013).

Finkelstein, V. (1996) *The disability movement has run out of steam. Disability Now* (February) 11.

Finkelstein, V. (2004) Representing disability, In Swain, J., French, S., Barnes, C. and Thomas, C. (Eds) *Disabling Barriers – Enabling Spaces* (second edition). London: Sage pp. 13–20.

France, F. E., Locock, L., Hunt, K., Ziebland, S., Field, K. and Wyke, S. (2012) Imagined futures: how experiential knowledge of disability affects parents decision making about fetal abnormality. *Health Expectations*, 15 (8), 139–156.

French, S. (Ed) (1994) *On Equal Terms: Working with Disabled People*. Oxford: Butterworth-Heinemann.

French, S. (2004) Can you see the rainbow? In Swain, J., Finkelstein, V., French, S. and Oliver, M. (Eds) *Disabling Barriers, Enabling Spaces*. London: Sage pp. 69–77.

Freund, P. (2001) Bodies, disability and spaces: the social model and disabling spatial organisations. *Disability and Society*, 16 (5), 689–706.

Gant, R. (1992) Transport for the disabled. *Geography*, 77 (1), 88–91.

Garland-Thomson, R. (1996) *Freakery: Cultural Spectacles of the Extraordinary Body*. London: New York University Press.

Garland-Thomson, R. (1997) *Extraordinary Bodies*. Chichester: Columbia University Press.

Garland-Thomson, R. (2002) The politics of staring. In Snyder, S., Brueggemann, B. J. and Garland-Thomson, R. (Eds) (2002) *Disability Studies: Enabling the Humanities*. New York: The Modern Language Association of America pp. 190–205.

Garland-Thomson, R. (2009) *Staring: How We Look*. Oxford: Oxford University Press.

Garthwaite, K. (2011) 'The language of shirkers and scroungers?' Talking about illness, disability and coalition welfare reform. *Disability and Society*, 26 (3), 369–372.

Gerber, D. (1993) Interpreting the freak and freak show. *Disability, Handicap and Society*, 8 (4), 435–436.

Gerbner, G. and Gross, L. (1974) *Trends in Network Television Drama and Viewer Conceptions of Social Relality, 1967-1973*. Violence Profile Number 6. Educational Resources Information Cente: Washington, DC.

Ghai, A. (2002) Disabled women: an excluded agenda for Indian feminism. *Hypathia*, 17 (3), 49–66.

Gignac, M. A. M. and Cott, C. (1998) A conceptual model of Independence anddependence for adults with chronic physical illness and disability. *Social Science and Medicine*, 47 (6), 739–753.

Gilderbloom, J. I. and Rosentraub, M. S. (1990) Creating the accessible city: proposals for providing housing and transportation for low income, elder and disabled people. *American Journal of Economics and Sociology*, 49 (3), 241–282.

Giroux, H. A. and Pollock, G. (2010) *The Mouse That Roared: Disney and the End of Innocence*. New York: Rowman & Littlefield.

Gleeson, B. (1997) Disability studies: a historical materialist view. *Disability and Society*, *12* (2), 179–202.

Gleeson, B. (1999a) *Geographies of Disability*. London: Routledge.

Gleeson, B. (1999b) Can technology overcome a disabling city? In Butler, R. and Parr, H. (Eds) *Mind and Body Spaces*. London: Routledge 98–118.

Gleeson, B. (2000) Enabling geography: exploring a new political ethical idea. *Ethics, Place and Environment*, *3* (1), 65–70.

Goffman, E. (1963) *Stigma*. London: Penguin.

Golledge, R. (1991) Tactual stripmaps as navigational aids. *Journal of Visual Impairment and Blindness*, *85* (7), 269–301.

Golledge, R. (1993) Geography and the disabled: a survey with special reference to vision impaired and blind populations. *Transactions of the Institute of British Geographers, New Series*, *18* (1), 63–85.

Good Access Guide (2002) Adjustments to the built environment. Available online: http://www.goodaccessguide.co.uk/dda/adjustments-to-built-environment.php (Accessed 06/12/2012).

Goodley, D. (2007) Towards socially just pedagogies: deleuzoguattarian critical disability studies. *International Journal of Inclusive Education*, *11* (3), 317–334.

Goodley, D. (2011) *Disability Studies: An Interdisciplinary Introduction*. London: Sage.

Goodley, D. and Runswick-Cole, K. (2012) The body as disability and possability: Theorising the 'leaking, lacking and excessive' bodies of disabled children, *Scandinavian Journal of Disability Research*, *15* (1), 1–19.

Government Equalities Office (2010) Equality Act 2010: what do I need to know? A summary guide to your rights. Available online: https://www.gov.uk/government/uploads/system/uploads/attachment_data/file/85017/individual-rights1.pdf (Accessed 30/08/2013).

Grosz, E. (1991) Freaks. *Social Semiotics*, *1* (2), 22–38.

Haberer, J. (2010) *The Little Difference: Dwarfism and the Media*. Norderstedt, Germany: Grin.

Hahn, H. (1986) Disability and the urban environment: a perspective on Los Angeles. *Environment and Planning D: Society and Space*, *4* (3), 273–288.

Hahn, H. (1996) Antidiscrimination laws and social research on disability: the minority group perspective. *Behavioral sciences and the Law*, *14* (1), 41–59.

Hall, E. (2000) 'Blood, brain and bones': taking the body seriously in the geography of health and impairment. *Area*, *32* (1), 21–29.

Hall, E. (2004) Social geographies of learning disability: narratives of exclusion and inclusion. *Area*, *36* (3), 298–306.

Hall, E. (2007) Creating spaces of well-being for people with learning disabilities. *New Zealand Geographer*, *63* (2), 130–134.

Hall, E. (2010) Spaces of wellbeing for people with learning disabilities. *Scottish Geographical Journal*, *126* (4), 275–284.

Hall, E. (2011) Shopping for support: personalisation and the new spaces and relations of commodified care for people with learning disabilities. *Social and Cultural Geography*, *12* (6), 589–603.

Hall, E. and Kearns, R. (2001) Making space for the 'intellectual' in geographies of disability. *Health and Place*, *7* (3), 237–246.

Haller, B. R. and Ralph, S. (2003) John Callahan's Pelswick cartoon and a new phase of disability humor. *Disability Studies Quarterly*, *23*(3). https://dsq-sds.org/article/view/431/608.

Haller, B. R. and Ralph, S. (2006) 'Are disabling images in advertising becoming bold and daring? An analysis of prominent themes in USA and UK campaigns' *Disability Studies Quarterly 26* (3). https://dsq-sds.org/article/view/716/893.

Halliday, J. (2011) *Life's too short sees audience shrink. The Guardian [online]*. Available online: https://www.theguardian.com/media/2011/nov/18/life-s-too-short-audience (accessed 14/4/2012).

Hansen, N. and Philo, C. (2007) The normality of doing things differently: bodies, spaces and disability geography. *Tijdschrift voor Economische en Sociale Geografie*, *98* (4), 493–506.

Hawksworth, M. (2001) Disabling spatialities and the regulation of a visible secret. *Urban Studies*, *38* (2), 299–311.

Heider, J. D., Scherer, R. C. and Edlund, J. E. (2013) Cultural stereotypes and personal beliefs about individuals with dwarfism. *The Journal of Social Psychology*, *153* (1), 80–97.

Herndon, A. (2002) Disparate but disabled: fat embodiment and disability studies. *NWSA Journal*, *14* (3), 120–138.

Hettrick, A. and Attig, D. (2009) Sitting pretty: fat bodies, classroom desks and academic excess. In Rothblum, E.Solovay, S. (Eds) *The Fat Studies Reader*. New York Press: New York. pp. 197–204.

Hinds, E. H., Motz, F. M. and Nelson, M. S. A. (2006) *Popular Culture: Theory and Methodology*. London: Wisconsin press.

Hine, J. (2016) Transport disadvantage and social exclusion in urban Scotland. *Built Environment*, *30* (2), 161–171.

Hine, J. and Mitchell, F. (2001) Better for everyone? Travel experiences and transport exclusion. *Urban Studies*, *38* (2), 319–322.

Holt, L. (2003) (Dis)abling children in primary school spaces-geographies of inclusion and exclusion, *Health & Place*, *9* (2), 119–128.

Holt, L. (2004) Childhood disability and ability: (Dis)ablist geographies of mainstream primary schools. *Disability Studies Quarterly*, *24* (3). https://dsq-sds.org/article/view/506.

Hopkins, P. (2008) Critical geographies of body size. *Geography Compass*, *2* (6), 2111–2126.

Hopkins, P. (2012) Everyday politics of fat. *Antipode*, *44* (4), 1227–1246.

Horton, W. A., Hall, J. A. and Hecht, J. T. (2007) Achondroplasia. *The Lancet*, *370* (9582), 162–172.

Hunt, P. (1966) *Stigma: The Experience of Disability*. Geoffrey Chapman: London.

Hunt, P. (1972) *Letter to The Guardian*. Available online: http://disability-studies.leeds.ac.uk/files/library/Hunt-Hunt-1.pdf (Accessed 26/05/2013).

Hunt, P. (1973) *Letter published in The Magic Carpet*. Available online: http://disability-studies.leeds.ac.uk/files/library/Hunt-Hunt-2.pdf (Accessed 26/05/2013).

Huff, L. J. (2009) Access to the sky: airplane seats and fat bodies, In Rothblum, E., and Solovay, S. (Eds) *The Fat Studies Reader*. New York: New York Press, pp. 176–186.

Hughes, B. and Paterson, K. (1997) The social model of disability and the disappearing body: towards a sociology of impairment. *Disability and Society*, *12* (3), 325–340.

imdb.com (2012) *Time Bandits*, imdb.com [online]. Available online: http://www.imdb.com/title/tt0081633/?ref_=sr_1 (Accessed 10/07/2012).

imdb.com (2020a) The Lord of the Rings, *imdb.com [online]*. Available online: https://www.imdb.com/title/tt0120737/Accessed (29/03/2020).

imdb.com (2020b) The Wolf of Wall Street, imdb.com [online]. Available online: https://www.imdb.com/title/tt0993846/ (Accessed 29/03/2020).

Imrie, R., (1996a) Abelist geographies, disablist spaces: towards a reconstruction of Golledge's 'Geography and the disabled.' *Transactions of the Institute of British Geographers, 21* (2), 397–403.

Imrie, R. (1996b) *Disability and the City.* Salisbury: The Baskerville Press.

Imrie, R. (1997) Challenging disabled people's access in the built environment: evidence from the United Kingdom. *Town Planning Review, 68* (4), 293–318.

Imrie, R. (1999) The body, disability and Le Corbusier's conception of the radiant environment, In Butler, R. and Parr, H. (Eds) *Mind and Body Spaces.* Abingdon: Routledge, pp. 25–45.

Imrie, R. (2000) Disability and discourses of mobility and movement. *Environment and Planning A, 32* (9), 1641–1656.

Imrie, R. (2004) From universal to inclusive design in the built environment, In Swain, J., French, S., Barnes, C. and Thomas, C. (Eds) *Disabling Barriers – Enabling Spaces* (second edition). London: Sage, pp. 279–284.

Imrie, R. (2012) Universalism, universal design and equitable access to the built environment *Disability and Rehabilitation, 34* (10), 873–882.

Imrie, R. and Edwards, C. (2007) The geographies of disability: reflections on the development of a sub-discipline. *Geography Compass, 1* (3), 623–640.

Imrie, R. and Hall, P. (2001) An exploration of disability and the development process. *Urban Studies, 38* (2), 333–350.

Imrie, R. and Kumar, M. (1998) Focusing on disability and access in the built environment. *Disability and Society, 13* (3), 357–374.

Imrie, R. and Wells, P. (1993) Disablism, planning and the built environment. *Environment and Planning C, 11* (2), 213–231.

Israel, M. and Hay, I. (2006) *Research Ethics for Social Scientists.* London: Sage.

Iwarsson, S. and Stahl, A. (2003) Accessibility, usability and universal design – Positioning and definition of concepts describing person-environment relationships. *Disability and Rehabilitation, 25* (2), 57–66.

Johnson, J. (2019) Cinema admission in the United Kingdom (UK) 2001-2019. *Statista [online].* Available online: https://www.statista.com/statistics/238215/cinema-admissions-in-the-uk/ (Accessed 24/04/2020).

Jolly, D. (2011) The billion pound welfare reform fraud: fit for work? Available online: http://disability-studies.leeds.ac.uk/files/library/jolly-The-Billion-Pound-Welfare-Reform-Fraud.pdf (Accessed 27/02/2014).

Karpf, A. (1988) *Doctoring the Media.* London: Routledge.

Kaufmann, P., Kuch, H., Neuhauser, C. and Webster, E. (2011) *Humiliation, Degradation, Dehumanization: Human Dignity Violated.* London: Springer.

Kearns, R. A. and Smith, C. J. (1994) Housing, homelessness and mental health: mapping agenda for geography inquiry. *The Professional Geographer, 46* (4), 418–424.

Keith, L. (1996) Encounters with strangers: the public's responses to disabled women and how this affects our sense of self, In Morris, J. (Ed) *Encounters with Strangers: Feminism and Disability.* London: The Women's Press, pp. 69–88.

Kennedy, D. (2003) *Little People*. Emmarus: Rodale.

Kirkland, A. (2008) Think of the hippopotamus: rights consciousness in the fat acceptance movement. *Law and Society Review, 42* (2), 397–432.

Kitchin, R. (1998) 'Out of place', 'knowing one's place': space, power and the exclusion of disabled people. *Disability and Society, 13* (3), 343–356.

Kitchin, R. (2000) The researched opinions on the research: disabled people and disability research. *Disability and Society, 15* (1), 25–47.

Kitchin, R. and Law, R. (2001) The socio-spatial construction of (In)accessible public toilets. *Urban Studies, 38* (2), 287–298.

Kitchin, R. and Wilton, R. (2000) Disability geography and ethics. *Ethics, Place and Environment, 3* (1), 61–65.

Kittay, E. F., Jennings, B. and Wasunna, A. A. (2005) Dependency, difference and the global ethic of longterm care. *The Journal of Political Philosophy, 13* (4), 443–469.

Kittay, E. F. (2011) The ethics of care, dependence and disability. *Ratio Jurnis, 24* (1), 49–58.

Kruse, R. (2002) Social spaces of little people: the experiences of the Jamisons. *Social and Cultural Geography, 3* (2), 175–191.

Kruse, R. (2003) Narrating Intersections of gender and dwarfism in everyday spaces. *The Canadian Geographer, 47* (4), 494–508.

Kruse, R. (2010) Placing little people: dwarfism and geographies of everyday life In V. Chouinard, E. Hall, and R. Wilton (Eds) *Towards Enabling Geographies.* Surrey: Ashgate, pp. 183–198.

Kvale, S. (2007) *Doing Interviews*. London: Sage.

Laurier, E. and Parr, H. (2000) Emotions in health and disability research. *Ethics, Place and Environment, 3* (1), 98–102.

Laws, G. (1994) Oppression, knowledge and the built environment. *Political Geography, 13* (1), 7–32.

Lefebvre, H. (1991) *The Production of Space*. Oxford: Blackwell.

Legislation.gov (2012) Equality Act 2010. Available online: http://www.legislation. gov.uk/ukpga/2010/15/section/6 (Accessed 27/05/2012).

Lenney, M. and Sercombe, H. (2002) 'Did you see that guy in the wheelchair down the pub?' Interactions across difference in public place. *Disability and Society, 17* (1), 5–18.

Lingsom, S. (2011) Public space and impairment: an introspective case study of disabling and enabling experiences, *Scandinavian Journal of Disability Research, 14* (4), 1–13.

Little People of America (2008) Frequently asked questions. Available online: http://www.lpaonline.org/faq- (Accessed 22/08/2013).

Loja, E., Costa, E. M., Hughes, B. and Menezes, I. (2013) Disability, embodiment and ableism: stories of resistance, *Disability and Society, 28* (2), 190–203.

Longhurst, R. (1997) (Dis)embodied geographies. *Progress in Human Geography, 21* (4), 486–501.

Longhurst, R. (2005) Fat bodies: developing geographical research agendas. *Progress in Human Geography, 29* (3), 247–259.

Longhurst, R. (2010) The disabling effects of fat: the emotional and material geographies of some women who live in Hamilton, New Zealand In Chouinard, V., Hall, E. and Wilton R. (Eds) *Towards Enabling Geographies*: Surrey: Ashgate, pp. 199–216.

Longmore, P. (2003) *Why I Burned My Books and Other Essays on Disability*. Philadelphia: Temple University Press.

Lovett, A. and Gatrell, A. (1988) The geography of Spina bifida in England and Wales. *Transactions of the Institute of British Geographers 13* (3), 288–302.

Macpherson, H. M. (2008) 'I don't know why they call it the Lake District they might as well call it the rock district!' The workings of humour and laughter in research with members of visually impaired walking groups. *Environment and Planning D, 26* (6), 1080–1095.

Macpherson, H. M. (2009) The inter-corporal emergence of landscape: negotiating sight, blindness and ideas of landscape in British countryside. *Environment and Planning A, 41* (5), 1042–1054.

Macpherson, H. M. (2011) Navigating a non-representational research landscape and representing 'under-represented groups': from complexity to strategic essentialism (and back). *Social and Cultural Geography, 12* (6), 544–548.

Martin, N. (2010) A preliminary study of broad disability related themes within the Edinburgh Festival Fringe. *Disability and Society, 25* (5), 539–548.

Massey, D. (1994) *Space, Place and Gender*. Polity Press: Cambridge.

Massie, P. J. Mayer, L. S. (2014) Bringing elsewhere home: a song of ice and fire's ethics of disability. In Fugelso, D. (Ed.) *Studies of Medievalism*. D.S. Brewer: Cambridge. pp. 45–49.

Matthews, M. H. and Vujakovic, P. (1995) Private worlds and public places: mapping the environmental values of wheelchair users. *Environment and Planning A, 25* (7), 1069–1083.

McDowell, L. (1999) *Gender, Identity and Place*. Oxford: Blackwell.

McRuer, R. (2006) Compulsory able-bodiedness and queer/disabled existence In Davis, L. (Ed) *The Disability Studies Reader*. New York: Routledge, pp. 301–308.

McRuer, R. and Wilkerson, A. (2003) Cripping the (queer) nation. *GLQ: Journal of Lesbian and Gay Studies, 9* (1–2), 1–23.

Meeuf, R. (2014) The nonnormative celebrity body and the meritocracy of the star system: constructing Peter Dinklage in entertainment journalism. *Journal of Communication Inquiry, 38* (3), 204–222.

Miceli, G. M. (2010) *The disavowal of the body as a source of inquiry in critical Disability Studies: the return of impairment? Critical Disability Discourse 2*, 1–14.

Milchalko, R. (1999) *The Two in One: Walking With Smokie, Walking With Blindness*. Philadelphia, PA: Temple University Press.

Milchalko, R. (2002) *The Difference That Disability Makes*. Philadelphia, PA: Temple University Press.

Milligan, C. (1999) Without these walls: a geography of mental ill health in a rural environment, In Butler R. and Parr H., (Eds) *Mind and Body Spaces: Geographies of Illness, Impairment and Disability*. London, Routledge.

Mock, S. (2020) "Against a dwarf": the medieval motif of the antagonistic dwarf and its role in contemporary literature and film. *Journal of Literary and Cultural Disability Studies, 14* (2), 155–170.

Morris, J. (1989) *Able Lives: Women's Experiences of Paralysis*. London: The Women's Press.

Morris, J. (1991) *Pride Against Prejudice*. London: The Women's Press.

Morris, J. (1992) Personal and political: a feminist perspective on researching physical disability. *Disability, Handicap and Society, 7* (2), 157–166.

Morris, J. (1995) Creating space for absent voices: disabled women's experiences of receiving assistance with daily living activities. *Feminist Review, 51* (1), 68–93.

Morris, J. (1996) *Encounters with Strangers*. London: The Women's Press.

Morris, J. (1999) The meaning of independent living in the 3rd Millennium. Available online: http://www.leeds.ac.uk/disability-studies/archiveuk/morris/The%20meaning %20of%20independent%20living%20in%20the%20new%20millenium.pdf (Accessed 19/07/2012).

Morris, J. (2001) Impairment and disability: constructing an ethics of care that promotes human rights. *Hypathia, 16* (4), 1–16.

Moshe, B. N. and Powell, W. J. J. (2007), Sign of our times? Revis(it)ing the international symbol of access. *Disability and Society, 22* (5), 489–505.

Moss, P. (1999) Autobiographical notes on chronic illness, In Butler, R. and Parr, H. (Eds) *Mind and Body Spaces*. London: Routledge 155–165.

Moss, P. and Dyck, I. (1996) Inquiry into the environment and body: women work and chronic illnesss. *Environment and Planning. D, Society and Space, 14* (6), 737–753.

Neuhauser, C. (2011) Humiliation: the collective dimension, In Kaufmann, P., Kuch, H., Neuhauser, C. and Webster, E. (Eds) *Humiliation, Degradation, Dehumanization: Human Dignity Violated*. London: Springer, pp. 21–36.

Norden, M. F. (1994) *The Cinema of Isolation: A History of Physical Disability in the Movies*. New Brunswick: Rutgers.

Nunkoosing, K. (2005) The problems with interviews. *Qualitative Health Research, 15* (5), 698–706.

Oakley, A. (1981) Interviewing women: a contradiction in terms, In Roberts, H. (Ed) *Doing Feminist Research*. London: Routledge, pp. 30–61.

Office of National Statistics (2019) How our internet activity has influenced the way we shop: October 2019. ONS [online]. Available online: https://www.ons.gov.uk/ businessindustryandtrade/retailindustry/articles/howourinternetactivityhasinfluen- cedthewayweshop/october2019 (Accessed 27/02/2020).

Øksenholt 2018 Øksenholt, K. V. and Aarhaug, J. (2018) Public transport and people with impairments – exploring non-use of public transport through the case of Oslo, Norway. *Disability and Society, 33* (8), 1280–1302.

Oliver, M. (1981) A new model of the social work role in relation to disability, In Campling, J. (Ed) *The Handicapped Person: A New Perspective for Social Workers* London: RADAR, pp. 19–32.

Oliver, M. (1989) Disability and dependency: a creation of industrial societies? In Barton, L. (Ed) *Disability and Dependency*. London: Falmer Press, pp. 7–22.

Oliver, M. (1990) *The Politics of Disablement*. London: Palgrave.

Oliver, M. (1994) Capitalism, disability and ideology: a materialist critique of the normalization principle. Available online: http://disability-studies.leeds.ac.uk/files/ library/Oliver-cap-dis-ideol.pdf (Accessed 19/06/2013).

Oliver, M. (1996) Defining impairment and disability, In Barnes, C. and Mercer, G. (Eds) *Exploring the Divide: Illness and Disability*. Leeds: Disability Press.

Oliver, M. (2004) The social model in action: if i had a hammer, In Barnes, C. and Mercer, G. (Eds) *Implementing the Social Model of Disability Theory and Research*. Leeds: The Disability Press, pp. 18–31.

Olney, F. M. and Brockelman, F. K. (2003) Out of the disability closet: strategic use of perception management by select university students with disabilities. *Disability and Society, 18* (1), 35–50.

Olsen, R. and Clarke, H. (2003) *Parenting and Disability: Disabled Parents' Experiences of Raising Children.* Bristol: Policy Press.

Olsvik, V. M. (2006) Vulnerable, exposed and invisible: a study of violence and abuse against women with physical disabilities. *Scandinavian Journal of Disability Research, 8* (2–3), 85–98.

Omansky, B. (2011) *Borderlands of Blindness.* London: Rienner.

Panero, J. and Zelnik, M. (1979) *Human Dimension & Interior Space: A Source Book of Design Reference Standards.* Whitney Library of Design: New York.

Park, D. C., Radford, J. P. and Vickers, M. H. (1998) Disability studies in human geography. *Progress in Human Geography, 22* (2), 208–233.

Parr, H. (1997) Mental health, public space, and the city: questions of individual and collective access. *Environment and Planning D: Society and Space, 15* (4), 435–454.

Parr, H., Philo, C. and Burns, N. (2004) Social geographies of rural mental health: experiencing inclusions and exclusions.*Transactions of the Institute of British Geographers, 29* (4), 401–419.

Patra, K. (2015) Super Bowl XLIX is the most-watched show in U.S. history. *NFL.com* [online]. Available online: https://www.nfl.com/news/super-bowl-xlix-is-most-watched-show-in-u-s-history-0ap3000000467823 (Accessed 27/2/2016).

Petrie, H., Darzentas, J. S. and Power, C. (2014) Self-service terminals for older and disabled users: attitudes of key stakeholders. In Miesenberger K., Fels D., Archambault D., Peňáz P., Zagler W. (Eds) *Computers Helping People with Special Needs. ICCHP 2014. Lecture Notes in Computer Science*, vol 8547. Springer, Cham. pp. 340–347.

Philo, C. (2005) The geography of mental health: an established field? *Current Opinion in Psychiatry, 18* (5), 585–591.

Philo, C., Parr, H. and Burns, N. (2005) "An oasis for us": In between spaces of training for people with mental health problems in the Scottish Highlands, *Geoforum, 36* (6), 778–791.

Porter, A. (2000) Playing the 'disabled role' in local travel. *Area, 32* (1), 41–48.

Priestley, M. (1998) Constructions and creations: idealism, materialism and disability theory, *Disability and Society, 13* (1), 75–94.

Pritchard, E. (2019) Hate speech and dwarfism: the influence of cultural representations, In Sherry, M., Olsen, T., Solstad Vedeler, J. and Eriksen, J. (Eds) *Disability Hate Speech: Social, Cultural and Political Contexts.* London: Routledge. pp. 116–128.

Pritchard, E. and Kruse, R. (2020) Introduction: cultural representations of dwarfism. *Journal of Literary and Cultural Disability Studies, 14* (2), 131–135.

Reeve, D. (2003) 'Encounters with strangers': psycho-emotional dimensions of disability in everyday life *Disability Studies: Theory, Policy and Practice.* Lancaster, UK: Lancaster University. 4–6 September.

Reeve, D. (2006) 'Am I a real disabled person or someone with a dodgy arm?': A discussion of psycho-emotional disablism and its contribution to identity constructions, paper presented at *Disability Studies: Research and Learning*, Lancaster, UK: Lancaster University, 18–20 September.

Reuters (2012) Tiny Lawyer sues witness. Times Live [online]. Available online: https://www.timeslive.co.za/news/world/2012-01-13-tiny-lawyer-sues-witness/ (Accessed 05/06/2019).

Reid, D. K., Hammond-Stoughton, E. and Smith, M. R. (2006) The humorous construction of disability. *Disability and Society, 21* (6), 629–643.

Rhodes, P., Nocon, A., Small, N. and Wright, J. (2008) Disability and identity: the challenge of epilepsy. *Disability and Society, 23* (4), 385–395.

Rock, P. J. (1988) Independence: what it means to six disabled people living in the community. *Disability, Handicap and Society 3* (1) 27–35.

Roulstone, A. (2004) Employment barriers and inclusive futures, In Swain, J., French, S., Barnes, C. and Thomas, C. (Eds) *Disabling Barriers – Enabling Environments* London: Sage, pp. 195–200.

Roulstone, A. (2006) Applying a barriers approach to monitoring disabled people's employment: implications for the Disability Discrimination Act 2005. *Disability and Society, 21* (2), 115–131.

Sancho, J. (2003) Disabling prejudice: attitudes towards disability and its portrayal on television. Available online: http://www.leeds.ac.uk/disability-studies/archiveuk/sancho/disability.pdf (Accessed 11/12/2012).

Sapey, B. (1995) Disabling homes: a study of the housing needs of disabled people in Cornwall. *Disability and Society, 10* (1), 71–86.

Sapey, B., Stewart, J. and Donaldson, G. (2005) Increases in wheelchair use and perceptions of disablement. *Disability and Society, 20* (5), 489–505.

Schanke, S. A. and Thorsen, K. (2014) A life-course perspective on stigma-handling: resilience in persons of restricted growth narrated in life histories. *Disability and Rehabilitation, 36* (17), 1464–1473.

Scheufele, D. A. and Tewksbury, D. (2007) Framing, agenda setting, and priming: the evolution of three media effects models. *Journal of Communication 57* (1), 9–20.

Schmelking, L. P. (1984) Hierarchy of preferences towards disabled groups: a re-analysis. *Perceptual and Motor Skills, 59* (1), 151–157.

Schwartz, D., Blue, E., McDonald, M., Giuliani, G., Weber, G., Seirup, H., Rose, R., Albuhoff, D., Rosenfeld, J. and Perkins, A. (2010) Dispelling stereotypes: promoting disability equality through film. *Disability and Society, 25* (7), 841–848.

Scully, J. L. (2010) 'Hidden labor: disabled/nondisabled encounters, agency and autonomy. *The International Journal of Feminist Approaches to Bioethics, 3* (2), 25–42.

Semonin, P. (1996) Monsters in the marketplace: the exhibition of human oddities in early modern England, In Garland-Thomson, R. (Ed) *Freakery: Cultural Spectacles of the Extraordinary Body*. London: New York University Press, pp. 69–82.

Shakespeare, T. (1994) Cultural representation of disabled people: dustbins for disavowal. *Disability and Society, 9* (3), 283–299.

Shakespeare, T. (1996) Disability, identity and difference, In Barnes, C. and Mercer, G. (Eds) *Exploring the Divide*. Leeds: The Disability Press, pp. 94–113.

Shakespeare, T. (1999) Joking A Part. *Body and Society, 5* (4), 47–52.

Shakespeare, T. (2000) Disabled sexuality towards rights and recognition. *Disability and Society, 18* (3), 159–166.

Shakespeare, T. (2004) Social models of disability and other life strategies. *Scandinavian Journal of Disability Research, 6* (1), 8–21.

Shakespeare, T. (2006) *Disability Rights and Wrong*. London: Routledge.

Shakespeare, T. (2013) The social model of disability, In Davies, L. (Eds) *The Disability Studies Reader*, Oxon: Routledge, pp. 266–273.

Shakespeare, T. and Watson, N. (1997) Defending the social model. *Disability and Society, 12* (2), 293–300.

Shakespeare, T. and Watson, N. (2002) The social model of disability: an outdated ideology? *Research in the Social Science and Disability*, 2 9–28.

Shakespeare, T., Wright, M. and Thompson, S. (2007) *A Small Matter of Equality: Living with Restricted Growth*. Newcastle: Newcastle University.

Shakespeare, T., Thompson, S. and Wright, M. (2010) No laughing matter: medical and social experiences of restricted growth. *Scandinavian Journal of Disability Research*, *12* (1), 19–31.

Sharpe, J. (2005) Geography and gender: feminist methodologies in collaboration and in the field. *Progress in Human Geography*, *29* (3), 304–309.

Shaw, F. E. (1979) Agenda-setting and mass communication theory. *International Communication Gazette*, *25* 96–105.

Shildrick, M. (2012) Critical disability studies: rethinking the conventions for the age of postmodernity, In Watson, N., Roulstone, A. and Thomas, C. (Eds) *Routledge Handbook of Disability Studies*. London: Routledge, pp. 30–41.

Shultz, K. and Germeroth, D. (1998) Should we laugh or should we cry? Callahan's humor as a tool to change societal attitudes toward disability. *Howard Journal of Communications*, *9* (3), 229–244.

Snyder, S., Brueggemann, B. J. and Garland-Thomson, R. (Eds) (2002) *Disability Studies: Enabling the Humanities*. New York: The Modern Language Association of America.

Soja, E. W. (1989) *Postmodern Geographies: The Reassertion of Spaces In Critical Social Theory*. London: Verso.

Solevag, A. R. (2020) Zacchaeus in the gospel of Luke: comic figure, sinner, and included "other". *Journal of Literary and Cultural Disability Studies*, *14* (2), 225–240.

Steinfeld, E. and Maisel, J. L. (2012) *Universal Design: Creating Inclusive Environments*. Hoboken: John Wiley and Sons.

Stewart, M. (2016) *Cash Not Care: The Planned Demolition of the Uk Welfare State*. London: New generation publishing.

Stone, S. D. (2005) Reactions to invisible disability: the experiences of young women survivors of hemorrhagic stroke. *Disability and Rehabilitation*, *27* (6), 293–304.

Sutherland, A. T. (1981) *Disabled We Stand*. London: Souvenir Press.

Swain, J. and French, S. (2000) An affirmation model of disability. *Disability and Society*, *15* (4), 569–582.

Taub, D. E., McLorg, P. A. and Fanflik, L. P. (2004) Stigma management strategies among women with physical disabilities: contrasting approaches of downplaying or claiming a disability status. *Deviant Behaviour*, *25* (2), 169–190.

Tepper, M. (2000) Sexuality and disability: the missing discourse of pleasure. *Sexuality and Disability*, *18* (4), 283–290.

Thomas, C. (1999) *Female Forms: Experiencing and Understanding Disability*. Buckingham: Open University Press.

Thomas, C. (2004) How is disability understood? An examination of sociological approaches. *Disability and Society*, *19* (6), 569–583.

Thomas, C. (2007) *Sociologies of Disability and Illness*. London: Palgrave Macmillan.

Thompson, S., Shakespeare, T. and Wright, M. (2008) Medical and social aspects of the life course for adults with skeletal dysplasia: a review of current knowledge. *Disability and Rehabilitation*, *30* (1), 1–12.

Tierney, S. (2001) A reluctance to be defined 'disabled'. How can the social model of disability enhance understanding of anorexia? *Disability and Society*, *16* (5), 749–764.

Tøssebro, J. (2004) Introduction to the special issue. *Scandinavian Journal of Disability Research*, *6* (1), 3–7.

Titchkosky, T. (2011) *The Question of Access: Disability, Space and Meaning*. London: University of Toronto Press.

Tregaskis, C. (2002) Social model theory: the story so far. *Disability and Society*, *17* (4), 457–470.

Tringo, J. L. (1970) The hierarchy of preference toward disability groups. *The Journal of Special Education*, *4* (3), 295–306.

Tyrrell, B. (2020) A world turned upside down: Hop-frog, freak shows, and representations of dwarfism. *Literary and Cultural Disability Studies*, *14* (2), 171–186.

Understanding Dwarfism (2013) *Basic facts about dwarfism*. Available online: http://www.udprogram.com/basic-facts (Accessed 09/01/2020).

Understanding Dwarfism (2012) Home page. Available online: http://www.understandingdwarfism.com/html/home.html (Accessed 14/06/2013).

UN General Assembly (2006) Convention on the rights of persons with disabilities. Available online: https://www.refworld.org/docid/45f973632.html (Accessed 17/01/2020).

UPIAS (1975) 'Fundamental principles of disability' Available online: http://www.leeds.ac.uk/disabilitystudies/archiveuk/UPIAS/fundamental%20principles.pdf (Accessed 12/02/2012).

Valentine, G. (2003) Geography and ethics: in pursuit of geography ethics and emotions in geography of health and disability research. *Progress in Human Geography*, *27* (3), 375–380.

Valentine, G. and Skelton, T. (2007) Re-defining norms: D/deaf young people's transitions to independence. *Sociological Review*, *55* (1), 104–123.

Vernon, A. (1996). A stranger in many camps: the experience of disabled black and ethnic minority women, In J. Morris, J. (Ed) *Encounters With Strangers: Feminism and Disability*. London: Women's Press.

Van Etten, A. M. (1988) *Dwarfs Don't Live in Doll Houses*. Rochester: Adaptive Living.

Vickerman, P. (2002) Perspectives on the training of physical education teachers for the inclusion of children with special educational needs - Is there an official line view? *The Bulletin of Physical Education*, *38* (2), 79–98.

Vickerman, P. (2012) Including children with special educational needs in physical education: has entitlement and accessibility been realised? *Disability and Society*, *27* (2), 249–262.

Vickerman, P. and Blundell, M. (2010) Hearing the voices of disabled students in higher education. *Disability and Society*, *25* (1), 21–32.

Vujakovic, P. and Matthews, H. M. (1994) Contorted, folded and torn: environmental values, cartographic representation and the politics of disability. *Disability and Society*, *9* (3), 359–374.

Walking With Giants Foundation, (2013) About primordial dwarfism. [online] Available online: http://www.walkingwithgiants.org/en/about-the-wwgf.html (Accessed 29/01/2013).

Warmsley, J. (1997) Including people with learning difficulties: theory and practice, In Barton, L. and Oliver, M. (Eds) *Disability Studies: Past, Present and Future*. Leeds: The Disability Press, pp. 62–77.

Wästerfors, D. (2020) *Required to be creative. Everyday ways for dealing with in-accessibility. Disability and Society*. [ahead of print].

Watson, A. (2019) Number of TV households worldwide from 2010 to 2018, *Statista [online]* Available online: https://www.statista.com/statistics/268695/number-of-tv-households-worldwide/ (Accessed 20/04/2020).

Watson, K. (2020) "With a smile and a song": representations of people with dwarfism in 1930s cinema. *Journal of Literary and Cultural Disability Studies, 14* (2), 137–153.

Watson, N. (2002) Well, I know this is going to sound very strange to you, but I don't see myself as a disabled person: identity and disability. *Disability and Society, 17* (5), 509–527.

Watson, N. (2004) The dialectics of disability: a social model of the 21st century? In Barnes, C. and Mercer, G. (Eds) *Implementing the Social Model of Disability Theory and Research.* Leeds: The Disability Press, pp. 101–117.

Wendell, S. (1989) Toward a feminist theory of disability. *Hypatia, 4* (2), 104–124.

Wendell, S. (1996) *The Rejected Body.* London: Routledge.

Wiesel, I., Bigby, C. and Carling-Jenkins, R. (2013) 'Do you think I am stupid?': Urban encounters between people with and without intellectual disability. *Urban Studies, 50* (12), 2391–2406.

Wilde, A. (2007) Are you sitting comfortably? Soap Operas, disability and audience Available from: http://disability-studies.leeds.ac.uk/files/library/wilde-Alison-Wilde-Dis-cover-2-Adapted-Paper.pdf (Accessed 01/06/2013).

Wilde, A. (2018) *Film, Comedy and Disability: Understanding Humour and Genre in Cinematic Constructions of Impairment and Disability.* London: Routledge.

Wilton, R. (2000) Grounding hierarchies of acceptance: the social construction of disability in Nimby conflicts.*Urban Geography, 21* (7), 586–608.

Wolbring, G. (2008) The politics of ableism.*Development, 51* 252–258.

Wolch, J. and Philo, C. (2000) From distributions of deviance to definitions of differencepast and future mental health geographies. *Health and Place, 6* (3), 137–157.

Woolf, J. (2019) *The Wonders: Lifting the Curtain on the Freak Show, Circus and Victorian Age.* Michael O'Mara Books: London.

World Health Organisation (2013) Disabilities. Available online: http://www.who.int/topics/disabilities/en (Accessed 30/08/2013).

Worth, N. (2008) The significance of the personal within disability geography. *Area, 40* (3), 306–314.

Worth, N. (2013) Visual impairment in the city: young people's social strategies for independent mobility. *Urban Studies, 50* (3), 574–586.

Index

For Product Safety Concerns and Information please contact our EU
representative GPSR@taylorandfrancis.com
Taylor & Francis Verlag GmbH, Kaufingerstraße 24, 80331 München, Germany

www.ingramcontent.com/pod-product-compliance
Lightning Source LLC
Chambersburg PA
CBHW070729220326
41598CB00024BA/3365

* 9 7 8 0 3 6 7 6 4 4 3 0 7 *